Journal of Health Politics, Policy and Law

Editor Eric M. Patashnik, Brown University

Associate Editors Nicholas Bagley, University of Michigan; Helen Levy, University of Michigan; Elizabeth Rigby, George Washington University

Book Review Editor Rick Mayes, University of Richmond

Special Section Editors Beneath the Surface: Joseph White, Case Western Reserve University; The Politics and Policy of Health Reform: Heather Howard, Princeton University, and Frank J. Thompson, Rutgers University

Social Media Editor Harold A. Pollack, University of Chicago

Managing Editor Jennifer N. Costanza

Former Editors Ralph A. Straetz, New York University; Theodore R. Marmor, Yale University; Lawrence D. Brown, Columbia University; James A. Morone, Brown University; Mark A. Peterson, University of California, Los Angeles; Mark Schlesinger, Yale University; Michael S. Sparer, Columbia University; Colleen M. Grogan, University of Chicago

Volume 42, Number 5, October 2017
Published by Duke University Press

T0369831

Contents

Special Issue
The Politics and Challenges of Achieving Health Equity

Special Issue Editors: Alan B. Cohen, Colleen M. Grogan, and Jedediah N. Horwitt

The Many Roads toward Achieving Health Equity
Alan B. Cohen, Colleen M. Grogan, and Jedediah N. Horwitt   739

Civil Rights and the Courts in Shaping Health Equity

The Role of Courts in Shaping Health Equity   *Mark A. Hall*   749

Viewing Health Equity through a Legal Lens: Title VI of the
1964 Civil Rights Act   *Sara Rosenbaum and Sara Schmucker*   771

Political Discourse and the Framing of Health Equity

Cancer and Race: What They Tell Us about the Emerging
Focus of Health Equity   *Keith Wailoo*   789

Framing Health Equity: US Health Disparities in Comparative
Perspective   *Julia F. Lynch and Isabel M. Perera*   803

Words and Deeds: Presidential Discussion of Minority Health,
Public Policies, and Minority Perceptions   *Daniel Q. Gillion*   841

How Health Policies Affect Health Equity

People, Places, Power: Medicaid Concentration and Local
Political Participation   *Jamila D. Michener*   865

Missed Opportunity? Leveraging Mobile Technology
to Reduce Racial Health Disparities   *Rashawn Ray,*
Abigail A. Sewell, Keon L. Gilbert, and Jennifer D. Roberts   901

How Immigration Policy Impacts Health Equity

Cautious Citizenship: The Deterring Effect of Immigration
Issue Salience on Health Care Use and Bureaucratic
Interactions among Latino US Citizens   *Francisco I. Pedraza,*
Vanessa Cruz Nichols, and Alana M. W. LeBrón   925

Falling through the Coverage Cracks: How Documentation
Status Minimizes Immigrants' Access to Health Care
Tiffany D. Joseph   961

Commentary

How the ACA Addressed Health Equity and What Repeal
Would Mean   *Colleen M. Grogan*   985

Health Equity in a Trump Administration   *Deborah Stone*   995

Introduction
The Many Roads toward Achieving Health Equity

Alan B. Cohen
Boston University

Colleen M. Grogan
University of Chicago

Jedediah N. Horwitt
Boston University

Abstract This special issue of the *Journal* is devoted to understanding the many roads that lead toward achieving health equity. The eleven articles in the issue portray an America that is struggling with the clash between its historical ideal of pursuing equality for all and its ambivalence toward achieving equity in all social domains, especially health. Organized in five sections, the issue contains articles that examine and analyze: the role of civil rights law and the courts in shaping health equity; the political discourse that has framed our understanding of health equity; health policies that affect health equity, such as the Medicaid program, as well as related strategies that might help to improve equity, such as the use of mobile technologies to empower individuals; immigration policies and practices that impact health equity in marginalized populations; and commentaries in the final section that explore how the Affordable Care Act has addressed health equity, how repeal of the law would jeopardize equity gains, and how the political discourse and culture of the Trump administration could adversely affect health equity.

Keywords health equity, health disparities, access to care, fairness

In a special issue whose title contains the phrase "Achieving Health Equity," it is most appropriate to begin by defining the term "health equity." How can we achieve something without first knowing what it is we are attempting to achieve? Although at first blush this intellectual activity seems straightforward, one quickly realizes the complexity involved. There are many definitions of health equity in the literature, a notable recent example is that of Paula Braveman (2014), who clearly distinguishes between the terms "health disparities" and "health equity." She

Journal of Health Politics, Policy and Law, Vol. 42, No. 5, October 2017
DOI 10.1215/03616878-3940414 © 2017 by Duke University Press

begins by using the Healthy People 2020 (CDC 2017) definition for health disparities:

> . . . a particular type of health difference that is closely linked with economic, social, or environmental disadvantage. Health disparities adversely affect groups of people who have systematically experienced greater social or economic obstacles to health based on their racial or ethnic group, religion, socioeconomic status, gender, age, or mental health; cognitive, sensory, or physical disability; sexual orientation or gender identity; geographic location; or other characteristics historically linked to discrimination or exclusion.

This definition makes clear that not all health differences should be defined as health disparities. In Braveman's view, and in our view in this volume, a *health disparity* is a health difference that is explained by social or economic factors other than illness, such as race, ethnicity, income, and education. Such disparities are unjust. We all are born with different health endowments and we make choices in life that impact our health along the way. However, when these endowments and choices, coupled with our experiences, are historically (and currently) linked to discrimination or exclusion, the observed differences in health raise issues about social justice. Indeed, this concern about social justice lies at the heart of the concept of health disparities (Braveman 2011, 2014).

It makes sense, then, that after years of documenting myriad health disparities based on race, ethnicity, gender, education, and socioeconomic status (Adler and Stewart 2010; Krieger 2001; WHO 2008), researchers, policy makers and advocates recently have shifted their focus from documenting the existence of disparities to addressing the underlying causes of those disparities. Indeed, the recent focus on *health equity* reflects growing interest in the social determinants of health and the pursuit of high-value health care in the United States (Adler et al. 2016; Betancourt 2016; Purnell et al. 2016; Thornton et al. 2016). It also represents a common goal to eliminate disparities in health. However, while this goal illustrates a consensus that health disparities are unjust and need to be addressed, it also likely masks policy disagreements regarding how to go about achieving health equity.

Braveman (2014) defines health equity as the pursuit of "striving for the highest possible standard of health for all people and giving special attention to the needs of those at greatest risk of poor health, based on social conditions" (p. 6). Although this definition offers some clarity, the term "possible standard" still allows for unequal distribution of health and raises the question (as we discuss below): How do we determine the highest possible standard of health? Moreover, it remains unclear what public policies or set of programs would bring us closer to achieving this goal. The lack of consensus stems not so much from an unresolved debate over the choice of solutions but rather from an implicit acknowledgment that many different approaches have been (and still could be) offered in service of achieving this goal.

For example, in attempting to attain the highest possible standard of health for all, some may argue that we need to focus on a model of patient engagement in which the patient is given full volition to pursue her own "highest possible standard of health" even if that results in an unequal distribution of health for all. This approach fits with the "process" view of equity (Nozick 1974), where the focus is on the fairness of the decision-making process, rather than the end result. Voting is a classic example of process equity: although only one person wins, people accept this result as fair and legitimate as long as the voting process is deemed fair. In contrast, others might argue that we should look at health outcomes (the end result) to determine if health equity has been achieved. What is important about the health domain is that although these two arguments are simultaneously in play, rarely are they ever debated as alternatives. Rather, complementary approaches to achieving health equity typically (and arguably must) happen across the divide between process and end results as well as across multiple levels of scale. The purpose of this special issue is to examine the broad array of approaches that have been attempted in the United States to address health equity through legal, social, and public health interventions, and to elucidate the political challenges that have affected how various policies—whether so intended or not—have resulted in better or worse health equity.

To illustrate this point we provide a conceptual framework that displays approaches to health equity across a process versus end results continuum (see fig. 1). As is the case in all countries, there are laws and regulations that dictate how providers deliver health care and how patients should be able to access care in a "fair" way. The term "fair" is in quotations because whether laws and regulations actually provide access to care in a fair way is subject to interpretation and therefore always contested. Contributors to this issue address different elements of process or end results within the framework.

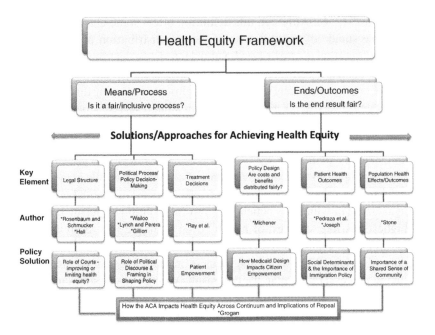

Figure 1 Health Equity Framework

In This Issue

The special issue is presented in five main sections. Articles in the first section examine the importance of civil rights and the role of the courts in shaping health equity. The second section contains three articles that document and analyze the political discourse that has framed our understanding of health equity and the policies that have been developed to address health disparities. The third section focuses on health policies that affect health equity, such as the Medicaid program, and on practical strategies that might help to achieve better equity, such as the use of mobile technologies to empower individuals. In the fourth section, two articles explore how immigration policy and practices impact health equity in marginalized populations. The issue concludes with two commentaries that analyze how the Affordable Care Act has addressed health equity, what repeal of the law would mean for equity, and how health equity will be affected more broadly by the political discourse and culture of the Trump administration.

We summarize here the salient points raised in the articles that follow. Looking back over the past fifty years, Mark Hall argues that the courts have played a limited, yet key, role in shaping health equity by impacting legal rulings and understandings in three main areas: racial discrimination, disability discrimination, and constitutional rights. Hall contends that the impact of the courts on health equity has been limited, largely because judicial enforcement has focused on overt, intentional discrimination in the delivery of health care, which is largely absent in the modern era. Thus far, the courts have been unwilling to use civil rights or constitutional law to address documentation of health disparities or of disparate impact by race or gender.

Sara Rosenbaum and Sara Schmucker focus specifically on Title VI of the Civil Rights Act of 1964, which prohibits discrimination by federally assisted entities on the basis of race, color, or national origin. Despite the major achievement of enforcing rapid desegregation of hospitals in the 1960s, a major limitation of Title VI has been the courts' refusal to apply the title to physicians, allowing them to remain free to refuse to accept particular patients. Rosenbaum and Schmucker also discuss the very important distinction between discriminatory impact and intentional discrimination, and the refusal of the courts to consider legal challenges to the former. Nonetheless, they conclude on a positive note, citing a recent resurgence to use Title VI to enforce basic compliance across a range of federally assisted programs. These two articles highlight the importance of having a strong legal framework in place to move the nation toward greater health equity.

Health equity also has been shaped historically through political discourse and the ways in which we have framed the issue itself. Using cancer care as a vehicle to illustrate his points, Keith Wailoo traces the transition of scholarly discourse from a focus on "health disparities" and "inequalities" to a more refined focus on "health equity." He argues that the shift is not purely semantic, but rather a political strategy to narrow the target of health reform efforts in the current era. Thus, he believes that the history of cancer and race may hold valuable lessons for the "long and winding road" of health reform related to improving health equity for all.

Julia Lynch and Isabel Perera explore the different conceptions of health equity in key national health policy documents in the United States, the United Kingdom, and France. They find substantial differences across the three countries in the characterization of group differences (by socioeconomic status or SES, race/ethnicity, or territory), and the underlying theorized causes of health inequalities (socioeconomic structures versus health care system features). Although reports in all three countries allude at least minimally to inequalities in social determinants as the underlying cause of health inequalities, the reports' authors stop well short of advocating the redistribution of power and resources that likely would be necessary to redress observed inequalities.

Examining the different rhetorical approaches used by US presidents since the 1960s to address minority health inequality, Daniel Gillion offers both a historical perspective and an empirical assessment of how that political discourse transported their discussion of minority health beyond the confines of Washington, DC, to local communities throughout the nation that had disproportionate numbers of blacks and Latinos. He finds that presidential discussion of minority health leads to greater salience on the issue and increases public health awareness. His work suggests that presidential messaging on minority health provides a framework for minority groups to understand and discuss the health disparities that may plague their communities.

The article by Jamila Michener focuses specifically on the political effects of concentrating Medicaid beneficiaries in particular locales. She first presents a framework for conceptualizing the community-wide consequences of policy concentration, and then analyzes aggregate longitudinal data to examine the effect of Medicaid density on county-level voter turnout and local organizational strength. Michener discovers that, as the proportion of county residents enrolled in Medicaid increases, the prevalence of civic and political membership associations declines and aggregate rates of voting decrease. Her findings suggest that, if grassroots political action is to be part of a strategy to achieve health equity, policy makers and local organizations must strive to counteract the demobilizing "place-based" political effects of "people-based" policies such as Medicaid.

Rashawn Ray and colleagues explore the potential for advances in technology to overcome racial barriers to health equity. Specifically, they examine how mobile online technologies may allow people to access and utilize health care in innovative ways. Using national survey data, they analyze racial differences in obtaining health information online via mobile devices, finding that blacks and Latinos are more likely than whites to trust online newspapers to get health information, and that minorities who have access to a mobile device are more likely to rely on the Internet for health information in a time of strong need. Federally insured individuals connected to mobile devices display the highest probability of relying on the Internet as a go-to source of health information. The authors conclude that mobile technologies may hold promise for helping to develop health literacy, improving health outcomes, and contributing to the reduction of health disparities by race and health insurance status.

Immigration policy and health policy have become increasingly intertwined in the twenty-first century, and there is growing evidence that health care utilization among Latino immigrants is adversely affected by restrictive immigration policy. Francisco Pedraza and colleagues investigate how immigration politics may negatively influence health care utilization among Latino US citizens, and the implication that health insurance expansions may not reduce health care inequities among Latinos who are concerned about exposure to immigration law enforcement authorities. Using data from the 2015 Latino National Health and Immigration Survey, they examine the extent to which the politics of immigration deters individuals from accessing health care providers and service-providing institutions. They find that Latino US citizens are less likely to make an appointment to see a health care provider when the issue of immigration is mentioned. Additionally, Latino US citizens who know someone who has been deported are more inclined to perceive that information shared with health care providers is not secure. The authors discuss how cautious citizenship or risk-avoidance behaviors toward public institutions in order to avoid scrutiny of citizenship status can be integrated into the formulation of policies aimed at reducing health care inequities.

Immigration policy also casts a shadow over recent health reforms. For example, most immigrants are excluded from the 2010 Affordable Care Act (ACA) owing to federal restrictions on public benefits for certain immigrants, but some states have extended coverage options to federally ineligible immigrants. In an examination of the relationship between coverage and health care access for immigrants under comprehensive health reform in the Boston metropolitan area, Tiffany Joseph finds that survey respondents across various stakeholder groups perceive that immigrants' documentation status minimizes their ability to access health care even when they have health coverage. Specifically, respondents express concern about the increased likelihood of deportation en route to medical appointments, which negatively influences immigrants' health care access. Thus, she believes that restrictive federal policies and national-level anti-immigrant sentiment can undermine inclusive subnational policies in socially progressive places.

In a concluding commentary, Colleen Grogan recounts the positive impacts of the ACA on achieving health equity and points to the dangers of repealing and replacing certain provisions of the law. It is no accident that the ACA explicitly mentions "health disparities" thirty-five times, or that all ten Titles of the Act contain efforts to reduce or eliminate such disparities. Although the ACA was not designed to overcome all health inequities, she explains how the specific provisions under each Title enable state and local governments, health care delivery programs, and providers—to name just a few of the actors—to put policies in place that begin the work of moving toward achieving health equity. Her analysis of the chief replacement bill, the American Health Care Act, indicates that, if passed by Congress, it will steer the nation further away from (rather than toward) achieving health equity.

In a companion perspective, Deborah Stone underscores the importance of equity as a political aspiration that transcends a philosophical standard for distributive justice. She presents strong arguments that equity can be sustained only through a culture of community in which people share an abiding sense of sameness and are actively willing to help other members of their community who are in need. She draws upon other articles in this issue to support her contention that the ACA's provisions regarding anti-discrimination must be preserved, and that the Trump administration and Congress should tread lightly when seeking to repeal and replace the ACA. Stone concludes by urging policy makers, policy analysts, and concerned citizens to resist policies that would undermine health equity and to remain focused on our national political and cultural institutions that make good policy possible.

Taken together, these eleven articles portray an America that is struggling with the disconnect between its historical ideal of pursuing equality for all and its demonstrated ambivalence toward achieving true equity in all social domains, especially health. Past failures to achieve health equity have been due, in part, to limitations in our laws and to unbalanced enforcement of those laws. But past efforts also have been limited by the restrictive ways in which health equity discussions have been framed and by health policies that, despite good intentions, have tended to be poorly designed and targeted for overcoming health inequities. Thus, there is a growing need to experiment with innovative strategies to improve health equity and, most importantly, to recognize and address the intersections that exist between health policies and other social policies, most notably immigration policy. As Colleen Grogan and Deborah Stone articulate in their commentaries, our nation is facing grave political challenges to our cultural institutions and our long-held ideals. The health equity gains achieved through ACA reforms are threatened by efforts to repeal and replace the law. While it is difficult to predict how events may unfold, it seems imperative that we rise to the stated challenges and muster the necessary political will to plot a clear course toward achieving health equity.

▪ ▪ ▪

Alan B. Cohen is a professor of health policy and management at Boston University's Questrom School of Business, and national program director of the Robert Wood Johnson Foundation Investigator Awards in Health Policy Research. He is the principal author of *Technology in American Health Care: Policy Directions for Effective Evaluation and Management* (Michigan, 2004), and coeditor of *Medicare and Medicaid at 50: America's Entitlement Programs in the Era of Affordable Care* (Oxford, 2015). A member of the National Academy of Social Insurance, he has published articles on health policy, comparative health care systems, quality improvement, and the rationing of care.

Colleen M. Grogan is a professor at the University of Chicago and academic director of the Graduate Program in Health Administration and Policy (GPHAP). Her research interests include health policy and health politics, the American welfare state, and participatory decision-making processes. She has written several book chapters, articles, and a co-authored book on the history and current politics of the US Medicaid program. She is currently working on a book titled *America's Hidden Health Care State*, which examines the intent behind America's submerged health care state. She is the former editor of the *Journal of Health Politics, Policy and Law*.

Jedediah N. Horwitt is deputy director of the Robert Wood Johnson Foundation Investigator Awards in Health Policy Research at Boston University. His areas of research include quality improvement, health information technology, hospital performance, global health investment and social lending, and infectious disease immunology. He has co-authored articles in the *Journal of the American College of Radiology*, *Medical Care Research and Review*, *American Journal of Medical Quality*, and *Immunogenetics*.

References

Adler, Nancy E., M. Maria Glymour, and Jonathan Fielding. 2016. "Addressing Social Determinants of Health and Health Inequalities." *Journal of the American Medical Association* 316, no. 16: 1641–42.

Adler, Nancy E., and Judith Stewart, eds. 2010. *The Biology of Disadvantage: Socioeconomic Status and Health*. Hoboken, NJ: John Wiley & Sons.

Betancourt, Joseph R. 2016. "Ushering in the New Era of Health Equity." Health Affairs Blog. http://healthaffairs.org/blog/2016/10/31/ushering-in-the-new-era-of-health-equity/ (accessed March 8, 2017).

Braveman, Paula. 2014. "What Are Health Disparities and Health Equity? We Need to Be Clear." *Public Health Reports*, supplement 2, 129: S5–S8.

Braveman, Paula A., Shiriki Kumanyika, Jonathan Fielding, Thomas LaVeist, Luisa N. Borrell, Ron Manderscheid, and Adewale Troutman. 2011. "Health Disparities and Health Equity: The Issue Is Justice." *American Journal of Public Health* 101, supplement 1: S149–S155.

CDC (Centers for Disease Control and Prevention). 2017. *Healthy People 2020.* https://www.healthypeople.gov/ (accessed March 8, 2017).

HealthyPeople.gov. "Disparities" http://www.healthypeople.gov/2020/about/disparities About.aspx (accessed November 20, 2012).

Krieger, Nancy 2001. "The Ostrich, the Albatross, and Public Health: An Eco-social Perspective—or Why an Explicit Focus on Health Consequences of Discrimination and Deprivation Is Vital for Good Science and Public Health Practice." *Public Health Reports* 116: 419–23.

Nozick, Robert. 1974. *Anarchy, State, and Utopia.* New York: Basic Books.

Purnell, Tanjala S., Elizabeth A. Calhoun, Sherita H. Golden, Jacqueline R. Halladay, Jessica L. Krok-Schoen, Bradley M. Appelhans, and Lisa S. Cooper. 2016. "Achieving Health Equity: Closing the Gaps in Health Care Disparities, Interventions, and Research." *Health Affairs* (Millwood) 35, no. 8: 1410–15.

Thornton, Rachel L., Crystal M. Glover, Crystal W. Cené, Deborah C. Glik, Jeffrey A. Henderson, and David R. Williams. 2016. "Evaluating Strategies for Reducing Health Disparities by Addressing the Social Determinants of Health." *Health Affairs* (Millwood) 35, no. 8: 1416–23.

WHO (World Health Organization, Commission on Social Determinants of Health). 2008. "Closing the Gap in a Generation: Health Equity through Action on the Social Determinants of Health." CSDH Final Report. Geneva: WHO.

The Role of Courts in Shaping Health Equity

Mark A. Hall
Wake Forest University

Abstract United States' courts have played a limited, yet key, role in shaping health equity in three areas of law: racial discrimination, disability discrimination, and constitutional rights. Executive and administrative action has been much more instrumental than judicial decisions in advancing racial equality in health care. Courts have been reluctant to intervene on racial justice because overt discrimination has largely disappeared, and the Supreme Court has interpreted civil rights laws in a fashion that restricts judicial authority to address more subtle or diffused forms of disparate impact. In contrast, courts have been more active in limiting disability discrimination by expanding the conditions that are considered disabling and by articulating and applying the operative concepts "reasonable accommodation" and "other qualified" in the context of both treatment and insurance coverage decisions. Finally, regarding constitutional rights, courts have had limited opportunity to intervene because, outside of specially protected arenas such as reproduction, constitutional law gives government wide discretion to define health and safety goals and methods. Thus, courts have had only a limited role in shaping health equity in the United States. It remains to be seen whether this will change under the Affordable Care Act or whatever health reform measure might replace it.

Keywords Civil rights, health equity, courts

Over the past fifty years, courts have played a limited, yet key, role in shaping health equity in the United States in three areas of law: racial discrimination, disability discrimination, and constitutional rights. In this article, I examine in various ways the roads courts have taken, the roads not taken, and possible future paths.

Journal of Health Politics, Policy and Law, Vol. 42, No. 5, October 2017
DOI 10.1215/03616878-3940432   © 2017 by Duke University Press

Racial Discrimination

Desegregating Hospitals

Despite the troubling racial disparities that exist in many areas of health care delivery, it is important to reflect on the substantial improvements in equitable access that occurred in prior generations. These improvements are largely attributable to the civil rights era, including its signature law, the Civil Rights Act of 1964. Prior to this law, at the end of the 1950s, most northern hospitals were integrated but almost no southern hospitals were (Reynolds 1997). Instead, in the South, hospitals almost uniformly either refused admission to blacks, sending them to separate, but definitively not equal, black-only facilities, or admitting them only to segregated wards. Even in the North, segregation existed in terms of medical staff membership. Most hospitals across the country would not accept African American interns or residents, and only a quarter would grant them staff privileges (Reynolds 1997).

By 1966, however, 85 percent of hospitals had desegregated and were no longer refusing black physicians (Reynolds 1997). Within a few additional years, overt racial discrimination among patients became unheard of. As the leading scholar summarizes (Smith 2015), within a remarkably short time span, US hospitals "went from the nation's most segregated private institutions to its most integrated." As Rosenbaum and Schmucker (2017) report in this issue, "intentional, legal segregation has disappeared from the scene of publicly funded programs and services."

These remarkable gains occurred mainly as a result of administrative actions and broader social movements, however, rather than resulting from court decisions. Whereas judicial leadership was needed to desegregate schools and other important social and government institutions, hospital integration occurred primarily as a result of regulatory and quasi-regulatory action. David Barton Smith recounts that, following the 1964 enactment of the Civil Rights Act, early enforcement efforts were targeted to southern hospitals. Building on that, Medicare's enactment in 1965 put pressure on all hospitals to comply with antidiscrimination norms that were imposed as a condition of hospitals' eligibility for Medicare funding. The Johnson administration's eagerness to ensure widespread hospital participation led it to enlist the support of the American Hospital Association (AHA) to convince member hospitals of the need to abandon past discriminatory practices. The AHA's supportive position also led to private enforcement of antidiscrimination standards through the Joint Commission on Hospital Accreditation.

Although administrative and accreditation authorities led the way to hospital desegregation in the 1960s, a key court decision helped to clear the path. Earlier federal law also prohibited racial discrimination by hospitals that had received construction funding from the Hill-Burton Act of 1946, but the enforcing agency maintained that "separate but equal" facilities constituted compliance. That position was successfully challenged in *Simkins v. Cone* (323 F.2d 959 [1963]), where the Fourth Circuit ruled that the government's separate-but-equal position was unconstitutional. When the Supreme Court declined to hear the case the following year, that action was widely viewed as endorsing the ruling. The prominence of this decision gave support to legislative efforts in Congress to adopt the Civil Rights Act soon thereafter.

Exempting Physicians and Disparate Impact

Following the rapid integration of hospitals in the 1960s, courts have not continued to open new routes for addressing racial discrimination in health care. Limited judicial action under the civil rights laws has been due in large part to the roadblocks established by the governing law and administrative interpretations, as detailed in Rosenbaum and Schmucker's article (2017). Principal among these has been the federal government's interpretation of Title VI of the Civil Rights Act that limits its application to physicians. Title VI prohibits discrimination based on "race, color, or national origin" by "any program or activity receiving federal financial assistance." Hospitals became subject to Title VI mainly due to Medicare and Medicaid funding, but the same has not been true for physicians. Federal agencies have consistently ruled that Medicare payments to physicians do not trigger application of Title VI because Part B of Medicare constitutes a "contract of insurance," which Title VI excludes from its definition of "financial assistance" (Crossley 2003). The same argument would not necessarily apply to Medicaid funding, but enforcement agencies failed to declare that Title VI applies to physicians who receive Medicaid funding, and the issue has not been litigated in court.

As a result, it has generally been assumed that physicians are free to discriminate on any basis they like due to the absence of express statutory authority stating otherwise (Orentlicher, Bobinski, and Hall 2013). *Walker v. Pierce* (560 F.2d 609 [4th Cir. 1977]), is a court decision that illustrates this gap in the law. There, two black female patients covered by Medicaid sued a South Carolina obstetrician for insisting that they be sterilized after delivering their children. The physician explained that, regardless of race, he had a personal policy of not treating women who refused to be sterilized after their third child if they "were unable to financially support themselves." The court ruled that there is "no reason why Dr. Pierce could not establish and pursue the policy he has publicly and freely announced. Nor are we cited to judicial precedent or statute inhibiting this personal economic philosophy."

The *Walker* case illustrates the extent to which patients are not protected from what are clearly inappropriate reasons for a physician to deny care. Although the physician's policy was targeted at women, no law at the time prohibited gender discrimination by physicians. And, although his policy likely had a disproportionate impact on blacks, civil rights laws still did not clearly apply — for reasons noted in the following section. In short, patients are not protected from morally problematic denials of care by physicians in the absence of a statute granting protection.

Judicial expansion of civil rights protections has also been blocked by a key Supreme Court decision regarding disparate impact. In *Alexander v. Sandoval* (532 U.S. 275 [2001]), the Court ruled that private parties may sue only for "disparate treatment," meaning intentional discrimination, but not for "disparate impact," which covers actions that, although neutral on their surface with regard to race, disproportionately affect minorities. The Court did not foreclose enforcement agencies taking action based on disparate impact, but it ruled that any agency regulations using that approach do not, in themselves, allow private enforcement using a disparate impact theory, and the statute itself allows private enforcement only for intentional discrimination. To date, the relevant enforcement agencies have not pursued disparate impact approaches in the health care arena.

A prominent example of this refusal to extend the reach of Title VI is the rejection of challenges to the location of health care facilities. When hospitals serving inner-city populations, for instance, were closed or moved to more affluent suburbs, lawsuits challenged those location or closure decisions based on the racial composition of the affected populations (Lado 1994; Watson 1990). Courts have consistently rejected these challenges, however, ruling that, absent actual discriminatory intent, merely a disparate impact on minorities does not constitute prohibited discrimination as long as the decision has a plausible, nondiscriminatory justification. See, for instance, *Bryan v. Koch* (627 F.2d 612 [2d Cir. 1980]; allowing closure of a public hospital in Harlem, for budgetary reasons) and *NAACP v. Wilmington Medical Center* (657 F.2d 1322 [3d Cir. 1981]; finding no discriminatory intent in the decision to relocate an inner-city Wilmington, DE, hospital to the suburbs).

Another path untaken relates to racial disparities in treatment. Voluminous evidence documents that blacks, as a group, consistently fail to receive the same level of care provided to whites across a broad range of conditions and treatments. Seldom, however, is this due to overt discrimination. Instead, divergent treatment patterns result from subtle forms of implicit or unconscious bias, as well as a variety of other socioeconomic factors that are not necessarily attributable to the care provider. No court decisions have yet considered whether disparate treatment patterns violate civil rights laws, but legal scholars believe that any such challenges would almost certainly fail under current law, again due to the absence of actual discriminatory intent (Crossley 2003; Matthew 2015).

Potential Changes under the ACA

Potentially, the Affordable Care Act, if it survives, would remove, or at least lower, several of these roadblocks to more expansive civil rights enforcement. Section 1557 of the ACA is a sweeping antidiscrimination provision that applies existing bodies of federal antidiscrimination law—covering race, sex, age, and disability, among other conditions—to any "health program or activity" that receives federal funding. Included are not only health care facilities, but also physicians and insurers. Discrimination is prohibited not only in the specific activity or program that receives federal funding, but also in any and all health-related activities conducted by these recipients of federal funding.

In its implementing rules, the US Department of Health and Human Services (HHS) has adopted some expansive positions that, if upheld by the courts and not undone by the Trump administration, go substantially beyond previous civil rights law (Benge 2016). Most significantly, the rule "interprets Section 1557 as authorizing a private right of action for claims of disparate impact discrimination on the basis of any of the criteria enumerated in the legislation" (81 Fed. Reg. 31375, May 18, 2016). Essentially, this reads the ACA as reversing the Supreme Court's *Alexander v. Sandoval* decision noted above. It can be expected that a ruling this bold will be challenged in court, but courts usually defer to an agency's interpretation of its own governing statute, if reasonable. Here, the agency noted that, although some parts of civil rights law previously did not allow private claims for disparate impact, other parts did, such as the law governing sex or age discrimination. The agency reasoned that, because section 1557 adopts a uniform nondiscrimination standard, it would not make sense to allow disparate impact claims for some forms of discrimination but not others. A different administration could take a different view, however.

A second potential expansion relates to coverage of physicians. Here, the agency's current rule is more equivocal. Without meaningful explanation, the agency declined to change its existing position that Medicare Part B payments do not constitute federal "financial assistance." This surprised some commentators who thought it was obvious that section 1557 reverses this long-standing omission. That omission was based in large part on the exclusion from Title VI of "contracts of insurance," but section 1557 explicitly includes insurance contracts; indeed, one of its main purposes is to apply discrimination law to the many private insurers that the ACA now funds. The agency briefly noted the existence of this and other arguments against its exclusion of Part B payments, but opaquely stated that it "does not believe that this rule is the appropriate vehicle to modify the Department's position."[1]

Nevertheless, the agency noted various expansive ways in which section 1557 covers physicians through other sources of federal funding. Most notably, the agency declared that participation in Medicaid constitutes "federal financial assistance," even though those funds are paid to physicians only by states. Federal enforcement agencies had not previously made a clear statement that Medicaid's form of indirect federal financing triggers federal discrimination law. Again, that ruling might be subject to challenge in court, or might be revisited if Medicaid is converted to more of a program of block grants to the states; if upheld, though, this position will substantially expand the potential scope of discrimination law enforcement in the future. Of greatest significance, combining the two areas of expansion noted here, it could become possible to argue that physicians violate discrimination law when, without good justification, they make different treatment recommendations for minorities than for whites, or for women than for men (Blake 2016; Steege 2011).

Disability Discrimination

Disability discrimination law is a second major area of civil rights legal protection. There are two central federal disability laws, § 504 of the

---

1. 81 Fed. Reg. 31375 (May 18, 2016). One possible basis for the agency's hesitancy is the historical background that President Johnson, in order to overcome physicians' opposition to Medicare's enactment, promised not to use Medicare funding as a basis for applying the newly enacted civil rights laws to physicians (Smith 2016). It obviously is debatable whether such a promise should still bind the government a half century later, but perhaps the agency did not want to resolve that particular question in the context of this rulemaking.

Rehabilitation Act of 1973, which governs federally funded programs, and the Americans with Disabilities Act of 1990 (ADA), which governs state and local programs and key aspects of the private sector (employers and "public accommodations"). Courts have been circumspect, but not entirely quiescent, in using these laws to shape decisions in two broad arenas: (1) medical treatment in individual cases, and (2) decisions about resource allocation in designing benefits covered by health insurance.

In brief summary, these laws prohibit discrimination on the basis of disability when the person in question is qualified for the service or program despite the disability, or when any disqualifying aspects of a disability can be overcome through "reasonable accommodations." Because *disability* is defined broadly in a manner that includes many medical conditions (such as having a chronic or infectious disease that limits a major life activity, *Bragdon v. Abbott*, 524 U.S. 624 [1998]), these laws have been used to challenge decisions relating to a variety of health conditions, made by both medical care providers and by health care insurers (public and private).

Like Title VI of the Civil Rights Act, the original disability law (the Rehabilitation Act of 1973) applied to only federally funded programs, and thus did not reach physicians. The ADA, however, overcame this limitation in 1990 by extending protections to all businesses and services available to the general public, which includes physicians in private practice. The ADA also covers both public and private insurers. Thus, this body of law has received more judicial development than has the more limited protection against racial discrimination.

Treatment Decisions

U.S. v. University Hospital (729 F.2d 144 [2d Cir. 1984]) is an early leading decision that wrestled with the extent to which these laws apply to medical treatment decisions. It involved an infant born with spina bifida—a severe birth defect in which the baby has a fully exposed spinal cord, an unusually small head, and excessive cranial fluid. At the time, the condition was often fatal and, even now, those who survive usually suffer from severe neurological and cognitive impairments. Based on prognosis, the parents declined aggressive treatment. The Reagan administration became interested in the case and requested records from the hospital. When it refused, legal proceedings ensued.

The federal circuit court upheld the hospital's refusal to submit to federal investigation, ruling that its decision not to overrule the parents' refusal of treatment did not constitute potential disability discrimination. The core rationale was that, even though Baby Jane Doe was obviously disabled, disability discrimination law scrutinizes denial of medical service only when that is done because of another disabling condition that is unrelated to the condition for which treatment is being sought. For instance, disability law would apply if a patient were denied a liver transplant simply because she is blind, but not if a liver transplant were denied to a chronic alcoholic or someone with a severe immune system disorder (even though these conditions are recognized disabilities).

The *University Hospital* court was concerned that discrimination on the basis of disability is much more complicated an issue than discrimination on the basis of race. Race is essentially never an acceptable basis on which to deny services, but in medicine it obviously is often acceptable and even desirable to make decisions based on the patient's full set of medical conditions. As the court noted, it is not easy to decide whether a denial of treatment is unfairly discriminatory or is based on legitimate consideration of the patient's disability: "It would invariably require lengthy litigation primarily involving conflicting expert testimony to determine whether a decision to treat, or not to treat, or to litigate or not to litigate, was based on a 'bona fide medical judgment,' however that phrase might be defined" (*U.S. v. University Hospital* [729 F. 2d 144]).

Thinking about these concerns, courts could take one of two positions. They could simply declare that disability discrimination law does not apply at all to medical treatment decisions, but that would not square easily with the statute's plain language or its legislative history. Instead, the *University Hospital* court limited application of these laws to "only where the individual's handicap is unrelated to, and thus improper to consideration of, the services in question." The distinction between conditions that are independent of the disability and those that are related is based on the ground that antidiscrimination law is designed to ensure that similarly situated persons receive the same treatment. When the need for treatment arises out of the disability, as when a severely disabled newborn needs a surgical procedure, there is no similarly situated person without the disability who needs the same surgical procedure.

The question shifts, then, to how exactly to interpret this concept of "relatedness." Because the human body is a highly integrated organism and not compartmentalized into relatively independent parts, a disabling illness generally has a wide-ranging effect on that person's needs for, or potential benefit from, medical treatment. Consider the example of HIV infection. Such patients may have higher risks of complications from any surgical procedure, but it is often feasible to accommodate that higher risk. What should a court do, however, if a medical provider would prefer not to undertake those efforts?

Glanz v. Vernick (756 F. Supp. 632 [D. Mass. 1991]) is an illustrative decision. The doctor refused to perform a simple procedure to alleviate a patient's earaches, stating that the patient's HIV infection posed too great a risk — both to the patient and the surgeon. The court ruled that this position "requires an individualized inquiry and appropriate findings of fact" about the surgeon's stated justification. Although the court noted that there is "some merit to the argument that the court should defer to a doctor's medical judgment, . . . [a]ccepting this argument at face value . . . would completely eviscerate [the law's] function of preventing discrimination against the disabled in the healthcare context. A strict rule of deference would enable doctors to offer merely pretextual medical opinions to cover up discriminatory decisions. The evidentiary approach [required] . . . properly balances deference to sound medical opinions with the need to detect discriminatory motives."

The Supreme Court endorsed this fact-based inquiry in *Bragdon v. Abbott* (524 U.S. 624 [1998]), a case in which a woman with HIV infection challenged her dentist's refusal to fill her cavity unless he performed the procedure in a hospital (she lacked insurance to pay for hospital-based dental work). The Court ruled that, in order for the dentist to insist on a hospital setting, he would need to show that office treatment posed "a significant risk to [his] health or safety . . . that cannot be eliminated by . . . provision of auxiliary aids or services." In assessing whether the dentist's fear of HIV transmission was objectively reasonable, "the views of public health authorities, such as the U.S. Public Health Service, CDC, and the National Institutes of Health, are of special weight and authority. The views of these organizations are not conclusive, however. A health care professional who disagrees with the prevailing medical consensus may refute it by citing a credible scientific basis for deviating from the accepted norm." On remand, the circuit court found in favor of the patient, based on evidence about the effectiveness of universal precautions to prevent transmission of HIV infection (*Abbott v. Bragdon* 163 F.3d 87 [1st Cir. 1998]).

Rather than refusing treatment outright, a provider might seek to refer a more difficult patient to a specialist whom the provider believes is better suited to meet the patient's needs. Referring patients poses similar issues about the reasonableness and evenhandedness of the provider's rationale, but the same court that decided the remand in the dentist case just mentioned later ruled that it would not closely scrutinize an obstetrician's decision to refer an HIV-infected pregnant woman to a specialized HIV pregnancy program for drug therapy designed to prevent transmission of HIV to the woman's child; see *Lesley v. Chie* (250 F.3d 47 [1st Cir. 2001]). Considering "the extent to which a court should defer to a physician's claim that he lacks the [necessary] experience, knowledge, or other prerequisites," the court found no legal violation, writing that, to prevail, a patient would need to show "the decision to be devoid of any reasonable medical support." "For example, a plaintiff may argue that her physician's decision was so unreasonable—in the sense of being arbitrary and capricious—as to imply that it was pretext for some discriminatory motive, such as animus, fear, or 'apathetic attitudes.'"

This court went on to explain, however, that "instead of arguing pretext, a plaintiff may argue that her physician's decision was discriminatory on its face, because it rested on stereotypes of the disabled rather than an individualized inquiry into the patient's condition." This effort to root out disability stereotypes contrasts with the *Walker v. Pierce* case above, which disturbingly upheld a physician's right to insist that two African American mothers be sterilized in order to accept them as Medicaid patients. When physicians adopt such racial stereotypes, they cannot currently be under federal discrimination law simply because the Civil Rights Act, unlike disability discrimination law, has not yet been applied to physicians in private practice.

Embedded in legal analyses of disability discrimination is the law's requirement to make "reasonable accommodations" that will avoid the need to refuse service. That concept too is challenging in the context of medical treatment decisions. Courts might say that if there are extra services that could improve a disabled person's ability to benefit, and the extra services are not too costly, they must be provided. Thus, if a person with a psychiatric illness needs a kidney transplant and psychiatric counseling would ensure that the patient complies with the medications and follow-up appointments, the clinic would have to provide the counseling.[2] But, what if the counseling does not appear to be working, or is only partially helpful?

A more expansive view of the law's purpose would emphasize the need to improve conditions for people with disabilities rather than simply avoiding discriminating against them. Thus, even though people with disabilities unavoidably may not benefit from medical treatment as much

2. This hypothetical is suggested by the facts of Payton v. Weaver (182 Cal. Rptr. 225 [Cal. Ct. App. 1982]), involving refusal to treat a dialysis patient who had behavioral problems that interfered with treatment. That case was decided under the state common law duty to not abandon patients, rather than under disability discrimination law, but the court's reasoning is illustrative. The court upheld the refusal to continue treatment because the physician did everything he reasonably could to attempt to improve the patient's behavioral issues.

as other persons, making reasonable accommodations might mean that we do not disfavor a person merely because their disability causes them to realize less benefit from treatment than other persons. These flexible and judgmental concepts are difficult to apply, however, and courts are reluctant to do so in ways that interfere with prevailing medical standards of care. As a result, courts so far have not been active in using disability discrimination law to scrutinize medical treatment decisions.

Insurance Coverage

Another arena where disability discrimination law potentially applies is the design of health insurance coverage, either public or private. Here, we consider not just whether a particular patient can benefit from a specific treatment. That might be the issue under a garden variety "medical necessity" dispute. Beyond that, we also consider whether disability discrimination occurs when health insurance designs its coverage in a manner that excludes or limits a category or class of treatments. For instance, insurance might limit or exclude what or when it pays for mental health care or for organ transplants. Such decisions can be based on both considerations of cost—how expensive it is to cover such treatments—and on medical need and benefit—that is, whether there are higher priorities to which limited resources should be devoted.

On this front, there are two leading Supreme Court cases. *Alexander v. Choate* (469 U.S. 287 [1985]) rejected a disability discrimination challenge to Tennessee's decision to limit its Medicaid coverage for hospitalization to a maximum of two weeks a year. The limit was imposed to help offset a budget deficit. The challengers objected that this limit would have a disproportionate impact on people with disabilities, who need more extended care. Acknowledging that the law does not require a showing of discriminatory animus, still, the Court sought to avoid an application of the law that "would in essence require each recipient of federal funds first to evaluate the effect on the handicapped of every proposed action that might touch the interests of the handicapped, and then to consider alternatives for achieving the same objectives with less severe disadvantage to the handicapped. The formalization and policing of this process could lead to a wholly unwieldy administrative and adjudicative burden."

The Court thus rejected the discrimination challenge, reasoning in part that the two-week limit is "neutral on its face [in that it] does not distinguish . . . on the basis of any test, judgment, or trait that the handicapped as a class are less capable of meeting or less likely of having. . . . [Instead, the] reduction in inpatient coverage will leave both handicapped and non-handicapped Medicaid users with identical and effective hospital services fully available for their use, with both classes of users subject to the same durational limitation." The Court also rejected any notion that states must alter their Medicaid benefits "to meet the reality that the handicapped have greater medical needs. To conclude otherwise would be to find that the [law] requires states to view certain illnesses, that is, those particularly affecting the handicapped, as more important than others and more worthy of cure through government subsidization."

In contrast, in *Olmstead v. L.C.* (527 U.S. 581 [1999]), the Court found a potential ADA violation where a state Medicaid plan covered long-term hospitalization for mental illness but not less restrictive community placement options. The Court reasoned that these patients could be "reasonably accommodated" if the state could expand its coverage without straining the budget for other mental health services. Going even further, *Lovell v. Chandler* (303 F.3d 1039 [9th Cir. 2002]) found an ADA violation where the state expanded eligibility for Medicaid up to three times the poverty level but excluded disabled participants from the increased eligibility parameters, even though the state said this was all it could afford.

Olmstead reached a different result than *Choate* mainly because the restriction in *Olmstead* targeted a class of patients essentially all of whom were disabled (those with mental illness serious enough to require hospitalization); thus, it was a case of discriminatory treatment rather than merely disparate impact. But what about programs that limit mental health treatment more generally or broadly? In *Choate* the Supreme Court cited approvingly a second circuit opinion holding that a broad limitation of mental health coverage does not constitute disability discrimination. The ostensible reason is that, although some mental illness is severe enough to be disabling, not all mental illness is such, and thus limiting all such treatment is neutral with regard to disability, even though a broad-based limitation might have a disproportionate impact on those with mental or emotional disabilities.[3]

Going even further, *Modderno v. King* (82 F.3d 1059 [D.C. Cir. 1996]) ruled that lesser coverage of mental health treatment is not disability discrimination because to rule otherwise would be "to invite challenges to virtually every exercise of the [insurer's or employer's] discretion with

---

3. See also *Saks v. Franklin Covey Co.* (316 F.3d 337 [2d Cir. 2003]; exclusion of fertility treatment such as in vitro fertilization does not constitute either gender or disability discrimination because infertility is not always a disability, and the plan excluded fertility treatment for both men and women).

respect to the allocation of benefits amongst an encyclopedia of illnesses."[4] And, in *Doe v. Mutual of Omaha Insurance Company* (179 F.3d 557 [7th Cir. 1999]), the court upheld a specific cap on treatment of AIDS-related conditions that limited coverage to just $25,000, noting that, if it were to strike this cap, then some equally or more serious diseases could still be capped but others not, according arbitrarily to whether or not the disease happens to entail a disability. On the other hand, *Henderson v. Bodine Aluminum* (70 F.3d 958 [8th Cir. 1995]) ruled that denying coverage for expensive new therapy for breast cancer is potentially discriminatory where the plan covered this treatment for other cancers and there is evidence that it works for breast cancer.

In sum, disability discrimination law, like racial discrimination law, primarily targets differentiation that is expressly based on the protected trait, rather than decisions neutral on their face that have a disparate impact on the protected group. For racial discrimination, this is a major limitation in the law because policies rarely differentiate based on skin color, ethnicity, or the like. However, under disability discrimination law, cases of explicit differentiation arise more frequently because the criteria used to define disability are often ones that have relevance for medical decisions.

Reconciling Competing Goals

Clearly, the operative concepts here are difficult for courts to apply. Moreover, they appear to lead to potentially perverse results for broader health policy. According to one law professor (Crossley 1995), "The ADA is an inadequate and even inept tool for resolving whether we should tolerate cost-conscious [insurance] policies" because its concepts are so poorly suited for articulating and understanding the underlying social policy debate.

Recognizing large scale that, in a world of limited resources, some limits on coverage are inevitable, the fundamental issue is how such "rationing" should be done. Setting fewer limits means that more people will be entirely uninsured, leading to more disability or less treatment of disability overall. Setting some limits thus can make treatment more available generally, both for those with and without disabilities. But, if limits are set coarsely, without regard to medical condition, then such "meat ax" limits receive less or no scrutiny under disability law, because they are viewed as more neutral.

---

4. See also Lenox v. Healthwise of Kentucky (149 F.3d 453 [6th Cir. 1998]; no ADA violation in excluding coverage for heart transplants).

More refined criteria for setting limits, however, run a greater risk of encountering discrimination scrutiny, for the very reason that they include more medical specificity. If allocation criteria are specified that are unrelated to disabling conditions, then discrimination law does not come into play, but it is difficult, perhaps impossible, for rational allocation criteria in health care to entirely avoid addressing medical criteria of need, risk, and benefit without including some criteria that relate directly to disability broadly defined. The same can also be true for other legally protected criteria such as age or gender. When that occurs, courts face the daunting challenge of deciding when such criteria are and are not appropriate.

Against this backdrop of uncertainty, consider how much clarity there is in the ACA's legislative language that forbids designing "benefits in ways that discriminate against individuals because of their age, disability, or expected length of life," or that are "subject to denial . . . on the basis of the individuals' . . . present or predicted disability, degree of medical dependency, or quality of life." This appears aimed at prohibiting the government's use of more refined health policy concepts such as "quality-adjusted life years" (or QALYs) to define the standard set of "essential health benefits" that private insurers must cover (in the individual and small group markets). However, another ACA provision says that "nothing . . . shall be construed to prohibit . . . [health insurers] from carrying out utilization management techniques that are commonly used as of the date of enactment of this Act." Undoubtedly, these concepts and their competing objectives will continue to challenge courts and administrative agencies for decades to come.

Constitutional Protections

So far, we have reviewed only statutory or regulatory protections. More fundamental are the civil rights protections built into the US Constitution. Here, the focus expands from protecting rights *in* health care to also protecting rights *to* health care. How patients are treated within the health care system is important, but perhaps more important is whether people have access to any kind of health care. Constitutional doctrine potentially addresses both dimensions of individual rights.

Constitution-Free Zone

Much of health law is a constitution-free zone, meaning that, so far as the federal Constitution is concerned, lawmakers are not required to protect or advance health, nor are they constrained, for the most part, in how they choose to go about doing so. This broad statement is subject to several very important qualifications—relating to procedural due process and to specially protected privacy interests, among other doctrines—but, these exceptions aside, the US Constitution is silent about health, which leaves lawmakers free to do just about anything they want or nothing at all. For a time, there was thought that *Roe v. Wade* (410 U.S. 113 [1973]), could expand into a more generalized constitutional freedom in important medical decision making, because that decision stressed the freedom of doctors and patients to exercise medical judgment without state interference when fetuses are nonviable. Subsequent abortion decisions, however, have phrased the protected right solely in terms of the woman's individual interest in avoiding procreation.

Most government positions on health care are easily justified under the Constitution because the Constitution has no general protection for individuals' "pursuit of health." As constitutional lawyers put it, our Bill of Rights is a charter of negative, not positive, liberties, meaning that the government constitutionally owes us nothing as long as it leaves us alone (*DeShaney v. Winnebago County Department of Social Services*, 489 U.S. 189 [1989]). *Wideman v. Shallowford Community Hospital* (826 F.2d 1030 [11th Cir. 1987]) provides a good example of this reasoning. There, a county ambulance service took a woman in labor to its preferred hospital rather than to the hospital where the woman's obstetrician was to meet her, resulting in a delay in care that the woman claimed caused the death of her infant child. The court rejected any claim based on denial of constitutional rights because the county did not owe any obligation to transport her at all; therefore, it cannot be held responsible for transporting her to the wrong hospital.

This case was argued under the constitutional doctrine of "due process." Also potentially relevant is the doctrine of "equal protection." Without turning this summary into a constitutional treatise, it is helpful to sketch these basic constitutional concepts. In the early part of the last century, the Supreme Court took an "activist" approach to reviewing the constitutional validity of state economic and social regulation under the due process clause. In *Lochner v. New York* (198 U.S. 45 [1905]), the Court struck down a state's regulation of maximum work hours as a violation of the fundamental right to contract. However, the onslaught of programs in the late 1930s designed to ameliorate the Depression caused the Court to retreat by substituting a more deferential, rational basis standard of review of state economic regulation. Thereafter, the *Lochner* era of "substantive" or "economic" due process was thoroughly repudiated as a valid form of judicial review for most social regulation. It survived only for legislation that affects special categories of "fundamental" interests or liberties.

Health laws can also be challenged under the equal protection clause, since they inevitably draw lines or distinctions between permitted and impermissible activities or actors. Any such class-based legislation will be reviewed under one of three standards: (1) suspect classifications (those based on race, for example, or those that intrude on other fundamental rights) will be subjected to strict scrutiny; (2) quasi-suspect classifications (such as gender) will receive intermediate scrutiny; and (3) all other legislative classifications will be reviewed under the rational basis standard. Because most health laws fall within this last, broad generic category of social and economic legislation, they usually receive only light constitutional scrutiny. States, may, for instance, draw fine and contentious distinctions, such as funding some abortions but not others (*Maher v. Roe*, 432 U.S. 464 [1977]; *Harris v. McRae*, 448 U.S. 297 [1980]), or permitting palliative care for a patient who refuses life support at the same time that the state criminalizes physician-assisted suicide (*Vacco v. Quill*, 521 U.S. 793 [1997]; *Washington v. Glucksberg*, 521 U.S. 702 [1997]).

Courts have been especially deferential to a state's power to protect public health. They have upheld states' public health actions so long as they are not "arbitrary" or "unreasonable" or "unnecessary" to protect public health. Thus, for instance, courts have upheld the constitutionality of every form of professional and facility licensure—from banning alternative practitioners to barring inefficient facilities.[5] Other, everyday health laws that have passed constitutional muster include those that require autopsies, that allow the removal of corneas for transplantation, and, most dramatically, that redefine the very essence of death, and therefore life (*State v. Powell*, 497 So. 2d 1188 [Fla. 1986]; *State v. Schaffer*, 574 P.2d 205 [1977]). Despite their obvious and sometimes profound impact on individual liberties, they require no extraordinary justification under prevailing constitutional analysis.

Instead of a sweeping right to pursue health, "fundamental rights" under current doctrine are limited to bodily integrity—that is, refusing unwanted treatment (e.g., *Cruzan v. Director, Missouri Department of Health*, 497

---

5. For example, see: Williamson v. Lee Optical of Oklahoma (348 U.S. 483, 485 [1955]); United States v. Rutherford (442 U.S. 544 [1979]); Sherman v. Cryns (786 N.E.2d 139 [Ill. 2003]); Mitchell v. Clayton (995 F.2d 772, 775–76 [7th Cir. 1993]); Albany Surgical, P.C. v. Georgia Dept. of Community Health (602 S.E.2d 648 [Ga. 2004]).

U.S. 261 [1990]), and certain specially protected "privacy" arenas such as procreation and parenting (*Griswold v. Connecticut*, 381 U.S. 479 [1965]; *Planned Parenthood of Southeastern Pa. v. Casey*, 505 U.S. 833 [1992]). In *Washington v. Glucksberg* (521 U.S. 702), the Court explained that, "in addition to the specific freedoms protected by the Bill of Rights, the 'liberty' specially protected by the due process clause includes the rights to marry, to have children, to direct the education and upbringing of one's children, to marital privacy, to use contraception, to bodily integrity, and to abortion. We have also assumed, and strongly suggested, that the due process clause protects the traditional right to refuse unwanted lifesaving medical treatment." Also, persons subjected to state confinement have special constitutional protections (*O'Connor v. Donaldson*, 422 U.S. 563 [1975]), and health laws can implicate the First Amendment right to the free exercise of religion, the Fourth Amendment right to be free from unreasonable searches and seizures, and the right to "just compensation" if the government takes private property (Hall 2009).

Despite this tapestry of protected arenas, coercive health laws that impinge these freedoms are often justified because they serve a compelling public interest and are narrowly tailored to meet that interest. Accordingly, courts have repeatedly upheld invasions of these strong substantive protections in order to promote either individual or public health. With appropriate safeguards, the government may, for instance, require small-pox vaccinations (despite the inevitable risks), commit psychiatric patients to forced treatment, force-feed comatose patients who have not clearly refused such treatment, quarantine people with infectious disease, or intervene surgically to save a full-term fetus.[6] In each instance, the justifications and analyses differ, and there are limits to what the government can require, but these precedents are notable for their permissive breadth.

Legislatures also gain considerable constitutional leeway when they condition government spending or privileges on obeying health policy requirements. Therefore, laws that might not be upheld standing alone are easily upheld if they are imposed as qualifications for receiving optional government benefits. On this basis, for instance, the federal government requires hospitals to treat emergency patients for free and it once forbade Planned Parenthood from discussing abortions (*Burditt v. U.S. Department of Health and Human Services*, 934 F.2d 1362 [5th Cir. 1991]; *Rust v. Sullivan*, 500 U.S. 173 [1991]). Similarly, there are no constitutional issues

---

6. See: Jacobson v. Commonwealth of Massachusetts, 197 U.S. 11 (1905); Washington v. Harper, 494 U.S. 210 (1990); Addington v. Texas, 441 U.S. 418 (1979).

created by setting Medicare rates too low,[7] and states can require doctors to accept Medicaid patients at reduced rates.[8]

Potential Constitutional Restrictions

Some conservative or libertarian justices and constitutional scholars call for fundamental change to this conventional constitutional regime. They would revive some version of the economic or substantive due process approach of the *Lochner* era by expanding the range of fundamental interests or tightening the justifications for restrictions of individual liberty. For instance, a panel of the DC Circuit sent shock waves through the health policy establishment with its 2006 decision in *Abigail Alliance v. Eschenbach* (445 F.3d 470 [D.C. Cir. 2006]), holding that the Food and Drug Administration (FDA) must make experimental drugs more readily available to terminally ill patients for whom there are no other therapeutic options. Two of the three judges reasoned that seeking medical treatment that might save one's life is a fundamental right, the restriction of which was not adequately justified here. The full court reversed this decision a year later, but the original decision still reverberates.

Legal scholars have also noted the Canadian Supreme Court's 2005 decision in *Chaoulli v. Quebec* (1 S.C.R. 791), striking down Quebec's ban on private health insurance that duplicates public coverage. Using reasoning under the Quebec Charter of Human Rights and Freedoms that broadly tracks US constitutional analysis under our Bill of Rights, the court reasoned similarly to the original *Abigail Alliance* decision that fundamental interests in pursuing health are at stake and that a sweeping ban on insurance is too broad.

Despite this noticeable undercurrent, substantial change in constitutional analysis of health care regulation is not likely to take hold in the United States any time soon. Only two of the DC Circuit Court's thirteen judges adhered to the original decision in *Abigail Alliance*, and the Canadian court's scrutiny under Quebec's Charter is much more aggressive than what one would expect under the US Constitution. As noted above, pursuing health has not been recognized as a fundamental right. Instead, US courts are inclined to characterize asserted rights in extreme or technical ways

---

7. See Nazareth Home of Franciscan Sisters v. Novello, 7 N.Y.3d 538 (N.Y. 2006); William Brewbaker, Health Care Price Controls and the Takings Clause, 21 Hastings Const. L. Q. 669 (1994).

8. See Dukakis v. Massachusetts Medical Society, 815 F.2d 790 (1st Cir. 1987); Downhour v. Somani, 85 F.3d 261 (6th Cir. 1996).

that tend to defeat their being constitutionalized. For instance, the medical-aid-dying case, *Washington v. Glucksberg* (521 U.S. 702), characterized the right at issue as receiving assistance in committing suicide, rather than choosing a humane manner to die. Similarly, the full court in *Abigail Alliance*, the cancer treatment case, characterized the right at stake as access to investigational drugs rather than pursuing all available means to avoid death. Despite inevitable shifts in the political and social views of the federal judiciary, there is not likely to be any fundamental reversal in these basic attitudes.

Those who might hope for more invigorated constitutional scrutiny of rights to health care should be cautious about the potential this might have to stymie government efforts to advance health policy goals. Constitutional rights can be a two-edged sword (or a two-direction shield). They not only can protect individuals from unfair treatment by government, they can also limit the range of actions that government may take. For instance, potential constitutional limitations arise under the First Amendment. In 2012, two different appellate courts ruled that the First Amendment limits requirements the FDA imposes in two prominent areas: (1) graphic warning labels on cigarette packages (*R.J. Reynolds Tobacco Co. v. U.S. Food & Drug Administration*, 696 F.3d 1205 [D.C. Cir. 2012]), and (2) restrictions on drug manufacturers' marketing of "off-label" uses of their products (*United States v. Caronia*, 703 F.3d 149 [2d Cir. 2012]).

These disputes have not yet reached the Supreme Court, but the potential for using the Constitution to restrict health policy is clearly seen in the Court's famous Affordable Care Act decision, *NFIB v. Sebelius* (132 S. Ct. 2566 [2012]). There, the law's "individual mandate" barely survived, but only because a majority of the Court ruled it is valid as a tax on a voluntary choice to be uninsured. On the other hand, a majority also ruled that the federal government may not require the purchase of insurance as a simple regulatory command. Whether that restriction impacts other important areas of health policy remains to be seen. But, even as a singular precedent, the Court's ACA case reminds us that, under long-prevailing doctrine, US constitutional law easily can do more to restrain than to promote equitable access to care.

Conclusion

This review demonstrates that courts have had only a limited role in shaping health equity in the United States. Across several bodies of law, the major achievement has been the rapid desegregation of hospitals in the

1960s, but that was attributable much more to administrative pressure under Medicare, as well as larger political and economic forces, than to judicial edicts under the Civil Rights Act. Otherwise, various civil rights protections, including disability discrimination laws, have had limited impact because the ability to seek judicial enforcement is strongest for overt, intentional discrimination, which is largely absent in health care in the modern era. The availability of judicial enforcement is much weaker for the forms of disparate impact that currently are more pervasive. And, constitutional rights have limited impact in health care beyond areas of special protections such as procreation.

It is open to debate whether or not these existing limitations in civil rights laws are inherent or might be subject to change. Wise health policy requires differentiating among patients, conditions, and treatments for various reasons. The core principle of equal protection is not only to treat like cases alike, but also to treat differences appropriately. Courts express reservations about using civil rights or constitutional law too aggressively to question professional and institutional decisions about which differentiations in health care are and are not appropriate.

Based on this reluctance, some legal and social scholars (e.g., Roberts 2013) believe that more progress toward health equity can be made by working outside of, rather than through, existing civil rights laws. Civil rights laws are well suited to protect against individual cases of invidious treatment. These laws are less well suited to producing more sweeping institutional and social changes, apart from overt segregation among patients, which has largely disappeared. Since the 1960s, broader health equity goals have been advanced much more by the introduction and expansion of health insurance and health care access programs that cover broad segments of the population than by enforcement of civil rights laws. For instance, when Medicare was first enacted, per capita medical spending for minorities was 26 percent less for hospital care, and 40 percent less for physician care, than spending for whites, but a generation later, per capita spending was substantially higher for minorities than for whites (Smith 2015).

This major correction came about not through civil rights laws, but by greatly increasing insurance coverage population-wide, which disproportionately benefits those who were most disadvantaged. Similarly, the Affordable Care Act's initial expansion of coverage and access, if sustained, would have much more positive impact on minorities than on the general population (Chen et al. 2016). In its first two years, the ACA produced insurance gains that were 50 to 100 percent greater among

Hispanics, blacks, Native Americans, and Asians than among whites (Tavernise and Gebeloff 2016). Also, the ACA's prohibition of medical underwriting and coverage of preexisting conditions directly benefited people with disabilities (Rosenbaum, Teitelbaum, and Hayes 2011).

Realizing these greater gains from lifting all boats should not deter us from vigilance in continued enforcement of antidiscrimination laws against intentional discrimination, wherever that exists. Nevertheless, efforts to use these laws to change the systemic effects of facially neutral policies might ultimately produce fewer gains than continued efforts to improve health care quality and access across the board.

▪ ▪ ▪

Mark A. Hall is the Fred and Elizabeth Turnage professor of law and public health at Wake Forest University, and a nonresident senior fellow at the Brookings Institution. He is currently engaged in research on health care reform, insurance regulation, and the doctor-patient relationship.
hallma@wfu.edu

Acknowledgments

I am grateful to David Orentlicher for permission to base the section on "Disability Discriminiation—Treatment Decisions" partially on unpublished materials that he originally wrote for the teacher's manual for our casebook (Hall, Bobinski, and Orentlicher 2013).

References

Benge, Spenser G. 2016. "Section 1557 of the Affordable Care Act: An Effective Means of Combatting Health Insurers' Discrimination against Individuals with HIV/AIDS?" *Indiana Health Law Review* 13, no. 1: 193.

Blake, Valarie K. 2016. "An Opening for Civil Rights in Health Insurance after the Affordable Care Act." *Boston College Journal of Law and Social Justice* 36: 235–86.

Chen, Jie, Arturo Vargas-Bustamante, Karoline Mortensen, and Alexander N. Ortega. 2016. "Racial and Ethnic Disparities in Health Care Access and Utilization under the Affordable Care Act." *Medical Care* 54, no. 2: 140–46.

Crossley, Mary A. 1995. "Medical Futility and Disability Discrimination." *Iowa Law Review* 81: 179.

Crossley, Mary A. 2003. "Infected Judgment: Legal Responses to Physician Bias." *Villanova Law Review* 48: 195.

Hall, Mark A. 2009. "The Constitutionality of Mandates to Purchase Health Insurance." O'Neill Health Law Institute, Georgetown University. http://scholarship .law.georgetown.edu/cgi/viewcontent.cgi?article=1020&context=ois_papers.

Hall, Mark A., Mary Anne Bobinski, and David Orentlicher. 2013. *Health Care Law and Ethics.* Frederick, MD: Wolters Kluwer.

Lado, Marianne. 1994. "Breaking the Barriers of Access to Health Care: A Discussion of the Role of Civil Rights Litigation." *Brooklyn Law Review* 60: 239.

Matthew, Dayna Bowen. 2015. *Just Medicine: A Cure for Racial Inequality in American Health Care.* New York: New York University Press.

Orentlicher, David, Mary Anne Bobinski, and Mark A. Hall. 2013. *Bioethics and Public Health Law.* Frederick, MD: Aspen.

Reynolds, P. Preston. 1997. "The Federal Government's Use of Title VI and Medicare to Racially Integrate Hospitals in the United States, 1963 through 1967." *American Journal of Public Health* 87, no. 11: 1850–58.

Roberts, Jessica L. 2013. "Health Law as Disability Rights Law." *Minnesota Law Review* 97: 1963–2035.

Rosenbaum, Sara, and Sara Schmucker. 2017. "Viewing Health Equity through a Legal Lens: Title VI of the 1964 Civil Rights Act." *Journal of Health Politics, Policy and Law* 42, no. 5: 771–88.

Rosenbaum, Sara J., Joel B. Teitelbaum, and Katherine J. Hayes. 2011. "The Essential Health Benefits Provisions of the Affordable Care Act: Implications for People with Disabilities." New York: Commonwealth Fund. /www.commonwealthfund.org /publications/issue-briefs/2011/mar/essential-health-benefits-provisions.

Smith, David Barton. 2015. "The 'Golden Rules' for Eliminating Disparities: Title VI, Medicare, and the Implementation of the Affordable Care Act." *Health Matrix* 25: 33–59.

Smith, David Barton. 2016. *The Power to Health: Civil Rights, Medicare and the Struggle to Transform America's Health Care System.* Nashville, TN: Vanderbilt University Press.

Steege, Sarah G. 2011. "Finding a Cure in the Courts: A Private Right of Action for Disparate Impact in Health Care." *Michigan Journal of Race and Law* 16: 439–69.

Tavernise, Sabrina, and Robert Gebeloff. 2016. "Immigrants, the Poor and Minorities Gain Sharply under Affordable Care Act." *New York Times*, April 17.

Watson, Sidney. 1990. "Reinvigorating Title VI: Defending Health Care Discrimination— It Shouldn't Be So Easy." *Fordham Law Review* 58: 939.

Viewing Health Equity through a Legal Lens: Title VI of the 1964 Civil Rights Act

Sara Rosenbaum
Sara Schmucker
George Washington University

Abstract Enacted as part of the watershed Civil Rights Act of 1964, Title VI prohibits discrimination by federally assisted entities on the basis of race, color, or national origin. Indeed, the law is as broad as federal funding across the full range of programs and services that affect health. Over the years, governmental enforcement efforts have waxed and waned, and private litigants have confronted barriers to directly invoking its protections. But Title VI endures as the formal mechanism by which the nation rejects discrimination within federally funded programs and services. Enforcement efforts confront problems of proof, remedies whose effectiveness may be blunted by underlying residential segregation patterns, and a judiciary closed to legal challenges focusing on discriminatory impact rather than intentional discrimination. But Title VI enforcement has experienced a resurgence, with strategies that seek to use the law as a basic compliance tool across the range of federally assisted programs. This resurgence reflects an enduring commitment to more equitable outcomes in federally funded programs that bear directly on community health, and it stands as a testament to the vital importance of a legal framework designed to move the nation toward greater health equity.

Keywords health equity, Civil Rights Act, Title VI

Introduction

Enacted as part of the watershed Civil Rights Act of 1964, Title VI prohibits discrimination on the basis of race, color, or national origin by both public and private entities that receive federal financial assistance. The aim of Title VI, a core part of a legal landmark in American history (Purdum 2014), is no less than to ensure that the vast machinery of federal social

Journal of Health Politics, Policy and Law, Vol. 42, No. 5, October 2017
DOI 10.1215/03616878-3940423   © 2017 by Duke University Press

welfare funding is used to reduce segregation and discrimination in all its forms, not enable it. As such, Title VI functions as a major policy lever for achieving fundamental change in the nation's social fabric. This overarching goal is to be accomplished through the establishment of formal, regulatory expectations on the part of the federal government not only that certain types of practices will cease but also that recipients of federal financial assistance will take affirmative steps to ensure that they administer their programs and services in a manner that promotes equality. Implicit in Title VI at the time of enactment was a further expectation that government efforts to end discrimination in federally funded programs and activities would be supplemented through private enforcement efforts; but a generation of shifting sands in judicial philosophy has considerably narrowed government's ability to rely on private enforcement efforts, thereby magnifying its own role in shaping Title VI as a legal framework for health equity.

Title VI was enacted at a time when legal segregation was still the norm in major sections of the nation. As racial segregation laws disappeared, the government interest in enforcement waned, although recent governmental use of the law as an instrument of change has regained considerable momentum. How to adapt a law such as Title VI to modern circumstances, however, emerges as a major issue. Like other civil rights laws grounded in the goal of racial justice, Title VI today confronts what perhaps might be characterized as a more pernicious problem: the residential segregation that affects minority Americans and is so closely associated with health inequity (Williams and Braboy Jackson 2005). Under such circumstances, the crucial legal question is the disparate racial impact of seemingly neutral laws. As a tool for addressing this form of discrimination, Title VI faces two basic challenges: problems of proof and the challenge of fashioning legal remedies that themselves do not cross racially impermissible lines under current judicial doctrine (i.e., quotas), while still addressing the racial effects of policies that produce a discriminatory impact. Nonetheless, Title VI represents a seminal achievement in the effort to reset the social compact, one whose terms remain highly relevant to today's challenges. To dwell simply on challenges of implementation and enforcement would be to miss the forest among the trees.

The Origins and Evolution of Title VI

As a central element of the 1964 Civil Rights Act, Title VI was a crowning achievement of the civil rights era that spanned from World War II through the 1960s, and health and health care figured prominently in its creation. Title VI was designed to serve a core purpose: to end discrimination based on race, color, or national origin within programs that receive "federal financial assistance."[1] Unlike Title II of the Act, which reaches purely private conduct by enterprises engaged in commerce (such as hotels, restaurants, movie theaters, and other places of public accommodation), Title VI rests on Congress's power—indeed, its constitutional duty as viewed by some legal observers and courts—to ensure that federal funding is not spent on private entities that discriminate (Abernathy 1981).

Title VI became law at a time when the desegregation of schools and other public services was a major focus of civil rights concern. Its underlying rationale rested in significant part on a decision by the United States Court of Appeals for the Fourth Circuit in *Simkins v. Moses H. Cone Memorial Hospital* (323 F.2d 959 [4th Cir. 1963] [en banc], *cert. den.*, 376 U.S. 938 [1964]). *Simkins*, which involved the denial of admitting privileges to black physicians and the admission of black patients by a hospital built with Hill-Burton funding, was an outgrowth of what David Barton Smith has termed 'The North Carolina Campaign,' a pivotal chapter in the history of the civil rights movement (Smith 1999). The *Simkins* decision emphasized the constitutional basis for barring the flow of federal funds to public or private entities that discriminated.

Indeed, revulsion over discriminatory practices in health care—what Martin Luther King Jr. termed one of the most "shocking and inhumane" aspects of racism—figured strongly in the Senate floor debate over passage (Smith 1999). At the time of enactment, the precise number of federally assisted health actors was not known with any degree of certainty (Abernathy 1981), although by 1963, when *Simkins* was decided, over 104 racially segregated hospitals had been built, the great majority of which were for whites only (Byrd and Clayton 2001). (As an aside, it is worth recalling that only one year later, the Johnson administration struck an agreement with the Senate—never codified in statute—to exempt physicians treating Medicare patients from Title VI [Smith 1999]. This agreement ostensibly rested on Medicare's original structure as indemnity insurance whose funds did not directly flow to physicians but instead were transferred to beneficiaries in repayment for the services they purchased.

---

1. The regulations define "federal financial assistance" to include: "(1) grants and loans of federal funds, (2) the grant or donation of federal property and interests in property, (3) the detail of federal personnel, (4) the sale and lease of, and permission to use, federal property or interest in such property without consideration or at a nominal consideration, and (5) any federal agreement, arrangement, or other contract which has as one of its purposes the provision of assistance." 45 C.F.R. § 80.13(f).

Today, most private physicians directly participate in one or more federal health care programs, which under § 1557 of the Affordable Care Act are now defined to encompass both insured and administered products offered by insurers that participate in federal programs.)

By its express statutory terms, Title VI prohibits acts of intentional discrimination by "any program or activity receiving federal financial assistance" (42 U.S.C. § 2000d). But the earliest implementing regulations, which remain in force today, go further, extending the law's prohibitions to conduct and practices that have the *effect* of discriminating. For example, regulations originally issued by the United States Department of Health, Education and Welfare following enactment—part of the government-wide rules that remain applicable today and touch virtually every form of federal financial assistance—outlaw "criteria or methods of administration which have the effect of subjecting individuals to discrimination on the basis of their race, color, or national origin," as well as practices that have "the effect of defeating or substantially impairing accomplishment of the objectives of the program [with] respect [to] individuals of a particular race, color, or national origin" (45 C.F.R. § 80.3[b][2]). Thus, Title VI rules, which endure today, establish two types of prohibited discrimination: (1) intentional discrimination, as measured by evidence pointing to a specific intent to exclude or segregate; and (2) policies or practices that may be facially neutral but discriminatory in impact (Perez 2002). Over the five decades of Title VI's existence, Congress has not refuted this far-reaching interpretation.

Title VI's prohibitions apply to any form of federal financial assistance, including grants, loans or contracts, other than "contracts of insurance or guarantee," which as § 1557 of the Affordable Care Act makes clear, do not include private health insurance coverage sold by entities that receive federal funding. Title VI also sweeps broadly in terms of the activities subject to its provisions, covering public and private actors alike. The statute defines the term *program or activity* to encompass all of the operations of state and local agencies receiving federal funding, governmental entities that distribute federal funds, colleges and universities, and private corporations or organizations engaged in education, health care, housing, or social services, or parks and recreation (42 U.S.C. § 2000d-4a). In other words, the receipt of federal funding by a governmental or private entity, or any part thereof, triggers a duty not to discriminate.

Title VI is, of course, a law and, by their very nature, laws can cast what many might prefer to think of as broader social matters in an uncomfortable light, opening up policies and practices to legal scrutiny, sanctions, and remedies for conduct and practices considered to come within their ambit. In no case is the desire to define a problem other than in legal terms more powerful than in the area of race discrimination: who possibly would want to equate regrettable social conditions with the legal concept of discrimination, particularly if no one is able to identify an overt legal practice (such as an ordinance that mandates segregation by race) that drives such results?

Not surprisingly, therefore, despite the underlying intent of Title VI, as legal segregation laws disappeared, so too the appetite for framing issues as discrimination inevitably diminished. Policies and practices that might, in fact, be contributing to racially identifiable results have been viewed as a problem that lay outside the purview of civil rights law. The concept of "disparities," used by minority health researchers to define the racially measurable impact of policies and practices, proved to be an easier way to maintain a discourse about race and society with those who would change the subject away from discrimination, conveniently overlooking the fact that Title VI was intended to reach both acts of deliberate segregation as well as practices that produced such effects. Indeed, the rise of disparities research, rather than propelling efforts to adapt Title VI to more modern conditions, may have provided a softer lens through which to view policies and practices that, in legal terms, would have been expressed as discriminatory in effect. For example, the failure of a hospital's surgeons to participate in Medicaid—disproportionately relied on by racial and ethnic minority groups—might produce disparities in terms of who has access to advanced surgical treatment. At the same time, a policy that extends admitting privileges to surgeons that refuse to participate in Medicaid might also be thought of as one that is discriminatory in effect.

By the early 1980s, Title VI enforcement already had been severely reduced. As David Barton Smith explains, the creation of an Office for Civil Rights within the United States Department of Health, Education and Welfare (later renamed Health and Human Services, or HHS) by the Nixon administration was actually an effort to separate civil rights enforcement from any direct connection to program operations and isolate it into a small, underfunded entity with no real powers (Smith 1999). Rather than elevating the cause, the establishment of a civil rights office was understood as designed to achieve precisely the opposite result (Smith 1999). The impact of this decision reverberated over decades. Civil rights enforcement staff disappeared, as did the office's budget, which lacked any separate funding for enforcement efforts (Rosenbaum and Teitelbaum 2003).

This governmental effort to move away from defining problems as ones covered by the broad reach of Title VI could be seen in the 1985 Report of the Secretary's Task Force on Black and Minority Health. Commissioned by the Reagan administration, the Report produced an extensive statistical compilation focusing on the excess rates of death and disability among racial and ethnic minorities. But as important as it was in advancing public understanding of the elevated risk of poor health and death among minority populations, the 1985 report also diverted the discussion away from a civil rights lens, presumably in order to make its findings more politically palatable. The Secretary's Task Force was chaired not by the director of the HHS Office for Civil Rights (who served as a member), but instead by a distinguished government health researcher (Dr. Thomas E. Malone). The Report contained no chapter on the status or potential relevance of civil rights enforcement; indeed, the Report contained no real discussion of the possible link between disparities on the one hand and the reach of Title VI into problems of disparate impact on the other. Instead, the Report tended to focus on chronicling racial differences rather than finding root causes of inequality. The Report offered recommendations for training more minority health professionals and for better health education for minority communities. But it was fundamentally devoid of an agenda for addressing discriminatory effects associated with facially neutral policies and practices, such as provider participation in public insurance programs, language barriers to health and social services, the siting and location of care, and the segregation of patients by payer source, which may have lacked any underlying discriminatory intent but nonetheless produced effects that disproportionately advantaged racially identifiable groups.

It would take many years for civil rights advocates to connect the findings from disparities research to the question of Title VI civil rights enforcement. The seminal Institute of Medicine study, *Unequal Treatment*, did a great deal to reframe research into health disparities as a source of evidence regarding racial inequality rather than mere racial differences. From this study has flowed something of a resurgence of governmental efforts to devise remedies that are grounded in concepts of overcoming inequality, which lies at the heart of Title VI, in order to address institutional policies and practices that have a discriminatory effect as well as those with discriminatory purpose. Chief among this reestablished link have been landmark policies, first introduced in 2000 under the Clinton administration, modified somewhat by the George W. Bush administration, and expanded under the Obama administration, to use the results of health disparities research as a means for establishing language access as a basic compliance requirement for federally assisted entities, ranging from health care programs to other programs receiving federal financial assistance and designed to address the broad range of social conditions that affect health.

Title VI: Covering the Breadth of Health Equity

Although health scholars often focus on the role of Title VI in the context of health care, Title VI has a panoramic scope, as broad as the range of federally assisted programs that bear on health equity. In both government enforcement and in efforts by private litigants to directly enforce its guarantees, the emphasis naturally has been on the regulations' effects test; that is, on policies and practices that appear to be associated with racially unequal results. This more modern use of Title VI offers insight into the comprehensive nature of the law's reach (Abernathy 2006).

Despite the context in which they arise, Title VI cases tend to focus on specific types of conduct: criteria or practices that make certain people less likely to qualify for assistance; practices that cause certain eligible persons to receive a lesser amount of assistance; practices that cause people to receive services of lower quality or in segregated settings; and practices that diminish or impair the value of the service. Furthermore, because Title VI applies government-wide, enforcement cases touch on virtually every federally assisted program or activity that bears on the health and well-being of the population, from education to mass transit, housing, child welfare, health care, and environmental health (Abernathy 2006; Edson 2004; Johnson 2014; Mank 2007; Yan 2013). As federal financial assistance has permeated the social fabric, so has the reach of Title VI.

As discussed at greater length below, in 2000 the United States Supreme Court ended the ability of private individuals to sue to enforce Title VI disparate impact standards. Prior to that point, private litigation strategies were frequently part of Title VI enforcement efforts. Some cases prevailed in court, others lost. More importantly, the filing of a case by private individuals served as a sort of strategic lever, encouraging plaintiff groups and public officials to negotiate solutions that could alleviate the discriminatory effects of policies and practices. Private litigation as an enforcement technique was used across many different social welfare spheres.

Beyond siting services, challenges have involved the use of eligibility or placement criteria that segregate racial minorities, or that deprive them of the value of the service or result in services of lower quality. In education, numerous claims have challenged the use of isolated IQ tests and other student placement tools that result in the concentration of minority children in programs and classrooms designed for those with limited intellectual ability (Abernathy 2006). Title VI also has been used to challenge nursing facility admissions practices that group all Medicaid beneficiaries in one wing of an institution, thereby effectively segregating black patients who disproportionately rely on Medicaid (Rosenbaum and Frankford 2012).

Title VI cases also have tested the impact of seemingly neutral program decisions to take a more expedient or less costly approach to a problem, such as condemning the land on which community gardens are flourishing in order to build new community housing, as opposed to acquiring other land at a somewhat higher cost that would leave community gardens intact (Abernathy 2006). The effects test cases also have involved practices or policies that appear facially neutral but that work to disfavor minority program beneficiaries, such as a decision by a public housing authority to give priority to rehabilitation services for homeowners as opposed to renters (Abernathy 2006). Title VI challenges also have tested the discriminatory effects of disciplinary actions by recipients of federal funding, such as school discipline (Johnson 2014), and actions by health care providers operating programs to treat substance use disorders and that report one group of patients to law enforcement (black pregnant patients exposed to crack cocaine), while not reporting other patients (white pregnant patients exposed to alcohol) (*Ferguson v. City of Charleston, South Carolina*, 186 F.3d 469 [4th Cir. 1999]).

Transit planning has received particular Title VI attention because of unusually creative advocacy work in the face of the extraordinary impact on minority communities that flows from the absence of public transit (Johnson 2014). Title VI cases have focused on the decisions by local and state transit authorities to upgrade transit options (such as fast airport rail service) used predominantly by white riders while relegating minority communities to limited and unreliable forms of transportation (Yan 2013). Most recently, residents of Baltimore challenged the governor's decision to divert transportation funding away from urban mass transit improvements in favor of highway investment (Complaint, *Baltimore Regional Initiative Developing Genuine Equality, Inc. v. State of Maryland, et al.*, DOT No. 2016-0059).

Title VI challenges have ebbed and flowed in their success. Since its inception, courts have accorded the statute an "an ancillary, but not co-equal, role in enforcing national antidiscrimination policy," waffling on whether Title VI should have a more or less stringent standard for discrimination than the Constitution (Abernathy 1981: 14). Challenges involving disparate treatment generally have more favorable outcomes for the plaintiffs because, where it can be proven that the defendant has plainly discriminatory motives, the matter not only clearly violates Title VI, but also the Constitution. The early Title VI school segregation cases provide examples of such obvious discriminatory behavior. Conversely, challenges alleging discriminatory impact have fared less well with federal courts since the statutory language does not define "discrimination" and much deference is given to agency guidance and findings on the matter. Challenges alleging discriminatory effects on the environment or transitory impacts have tended to have less successful outcomes for plaintiffs, because of the unwillingness on the part of the courts to develop complex remedies other than those created by an enforcement agency itself.

The Complexity of Title VI as a Tool to Achieve Health Equity

All legal actions are difficult; for several reasons, using Title VI may be especially complicated. The first reason might be thought of as one of framing. For perfectly understandable reasons, there is a resistance to labeling a particular policy or practice as one that may place it within the legal lexicon of a statute whose purpose is to address discrimination on the basis of race or national origin, especially practices and conduct that are seemingly neutral but that produce discriminatory effects. Policies that hurt the poor may be repugnant on many grounds, but should they be considered discriminatory because the poor are more likely to be members of racial or ethnic minority groups? Resistance to such characterization is inevitable, particularly in a nation whose very existence rests on the original sin of racism and classification and segregation based on race. If investing transit funds in commuter trains from the suburbs rather than subways in the inner city is viewed simply as government choice regarding resource allocation with adverse fallout on the poor, this essentially sidesteps the question of whether federally assisted entities should be viewed as having a duty to avoid such fallout when the poor are, in fact, racially identifiable. Many might prefer to address the solution as one of fairer economic investment rather than as one grounded in racial justice owing to generations of practices that have produced racially identifiable outcomes where income and wealth are concerned.

A second problem relates to the challenges of proving a claim and answering defenses. To show disparate impact, a challenger must demonstrate a nexus between a particular policy and racially identifiable effects. For example, requiring all nursing home residents covered by Medicaid to be housed in a separate wing may be repugnant social policy, but it becomes a Title VI matter only if it can be shown that Medicaid patients are disproportionately African American. But what happens when no data on the race of Medicaid patients are available? Federal programs require recipients of assistance to maintain substantial racial data on those who receive benefits, but certain situations may be more subtle, such as particular settings in which patients are seen (a private physician's office rather than a specialty residency rotation clinic), or a first-come-first-serve policy for obtaining certain benefits in communities in which it is harder for certain racially distinct groups of residents to either understand the policy or arrive early.

Furthermore, it may be necessary to show that the observed racial results rest on other, equally plausible explanations. For example, in health care, simply showing that minority cancer patients receive less advanced cancer treatments is not sufficient. The challenger also would have to demonstrate that minority patients are not offered certain choices and that, when given equal choice, minority patients are equally as likely to prefer more advanced care. While simulation studies conducted by researchers have, in fact, shown racial bias in diagnosing and treating patients (Schulman et al. 1999), this is not the same as proving in a judicial or administrative setting that a particular policy maintained by a particular health care institution resulted in less equitable treatment. In other words, law is quite specific, and a finding of discriminatory practices cannot rest on simulations (although simulation experiments certainly may be relevant in helping explain institutional behavior). That is to say, the presence of statistical disparities alone do not show that a policy or practice had a discriminatory effect. This does not mean that intentional discrimination must be proved, but it does mean that a challenger would need to draw a link between the statistical evidence and an actual policy or practice. Proof of this nature is time consuming and costly.

Additionally, a showing of discrimination may not be sufficient. There are defenses such as the necessity of certain policies even if they do have a discriminatory impact. Steps to mitigate the impact of such policies might be ordered, but the policies may survive essentially intact. For example, stopping a hospital from leaving a poor, heavily minority community and relocating to a more affluent service area is virtually impossible, even though federal regulations governing the application of Title VI to health care explicitly offer the example of hospital siting practices as one that may fall within the purview of the law. A court might order the hospital to open a satellite clinic in a poor neighborhood as well as free shuttle services to its main campus, but the hospital relocation itself moves forward (Rosenbaum and Frankford 2012).

A third problem relates to remedies: How far should the courts go in second-guessing the decisions of program administrators regarding resource allocation in the case of programs that are often seriously underfinanced and on a daily basis demand difficult decisions about priorities; and if imbalances are found, how far can the courts or agencies go in imposing affirmative balancing remedies?

The history of the Title VI effects test, not found in the statute but established by regulation, has been fraught with challenges. In *Lau v. Nichols* (414 U.S. 563 [1974]), a unanimous Supreme Court held that a recipient of federal financial assistance could be liable under the terms of Title VI (if not the Constitution itself) for practices that discriminated within the meaning of Act, in this case, the lack of language-accessible programs for San Francisco public school children of Asian descent. The lower court had rejected the children's claims, finding that their poverty, not actions on the part of the school system, was at fault. Reversing, the Court based its rulings on federal Title VI rules applicable to schools, which utilized an effects test and required educational programs to take affirmative steps to help students overcome language barriers. In this case, the San Francisco school system's failure to affirmatively help children overcome their language barriers violated the rules and "effectively foreclosed" such students from "any meaningful education" (*Lau*, 414 U.S., p. 566.). *Lau* represented the "high-water mark" in terms of the willingness of the judiciary to halt practices that, even if not intentional and thereby a direct violation of the Constitution, could be shown to have a discriminatory impact (Abernathy 1981: 17).

But the limits of Title VI from the Court's perspective became evident in *Regents of the University of California v. Bakke* (438 U.S. 265 [1978]), which involved the use of affirmative action tools by the University of California (specifically, racial quotas) to weigh medical school admission decisions. While *Bakke* did not overturn *Lau*, it signaled the Court's willingness to impose significant limits on the reach of Title VI's remedial powers beyond its basic constitutional underpinning of outlawing intentional segregation and discrimination by race. In so doing, the Court signaled a sharp constraint on the ability of federally assisted entities to devise remedies, in this case, quantifiable, to address race-specific measures of inclusiveness that exceeded constitutional constraints under the Fourteenth Amendment (Abernathy 1981; Johnson 2014). This question of how far government can go to remedy the past effects of discrimination in federally assisted programs, or to avert the possibility of racially unequal results, continues to dominate civil rights law to the present.

Beyond the constitutional constraints on remedies that turn on affirmative efforts to achieve equity through the use of quantifiable targets, the question of remedies under the Title VI effects test raises other issues. One review of Title VI cases concludes that, in the main, agencies and judges appreciate the difficult balancing decisions that go into the operation of federally assisted programs (Abernathy 2006). As a result, business necessity constitutes a recognized defense under Title VI (Watson 1990), and in reviewing the legality of agency practices, courts will look to their reasonableness, a standard of review substantially lower than the compelling interest standard needed to justify practices found to amount to intentional discrimination (Abernathy 2006). It is hard, in other words, to convince a court or an agency that a particular decision affecting programs and services operated for a large and diverse population must be reversed or modified based on evidence of impact on a subset, although it is by no means impossible, as is illustrated by numerous cases involving negotiated settlements softening or modifying policies and practices shown to have a disparate impact on minority populations (Johnson 2014; Rubin-Wills 2012; Yan 2013). For example, in hospital siting cases, settlements have involved the establishment of satellite services in communities losing access to the main hospital facility (Rosenbaum and Frankford 2012). Similarly, in transit cases, advocates have achieved significant modifications in regional transportation plans to ensure a more reasonable level of investment in minority communities (Johnson 2014; Yan 2013).

Finally is the question of who has the right to enforce Title VI's disparate impact prohibitions. Unlike Title VII of the 1964 Civil Rights Act, which bars discrimination on prohibited grounds in the case of employment, Title VI contains no express right to relief in the courts, a crucial issue in modern jurisprudence (Rosenbaum and Frankford 2012). In *Bakke*, which arose under Title VI and dates back to a time when the courts were less strict about clear evidence regarding the right of private individuals to seek judicial intervention under "implied right of action" theory, the United States Supreme Court essentially assumed such a right. But in *Alexander v. Sandoval* (532 U.S. 275 [2001]), a case in which private litigants challenged Alabama's policy of English-only drivers' license tests, the Court foreclosed private judicial actions to enforce the federal effects test rule, limiting access to the courts to claims of intentional discrimination brought directly under the statute (Abernathy 2006;

Harvard 2001; Johnson 2014; Perez 2002; Rosenbaum and Teitelbaum 2003). At least one scholar has argued that, in a health care context, the ACA's extension of Title VI protections to new insurance markets may restore a private right of action for violations of the Title VI disparate impact rules (Steege 2011). But this theory has not yet been tested. As one might imagine, the *Sandoval* decision was an enormous blow to private enforcement efforts under Title VI, made all the more necessary by under-resourced federal enforcement agencies hobbled in their work by the politics of discrimination oversight. Since the major thrust of efforts to use Title VI to secure more equitable treatment entailed reliance on disparate impact theory, the loss of access to the courts has posed significant problems.

In fact, however, *Sandoval* also helped trigger a flowering of other strategies, including an increase in the use of federal administrative complaints by private individuals, and more importantly perhaps, efforts by government itself to build tests of equity into federal financial assistance through the use of clear, measurable, and prospective compliance standards embedded directly into regulatory standards. Indeed, one could argue that *Sandoval* effectively caused the federal agencies to do what they were supposed to do in the beginning, namely, make equitable conduct an explicit part of the operation of federally assisted programs. The HHS language access standards offer a crucial illustration of clear and measurable standards that are designed to act as a standard of Title VI compliance for federally assisted entities. Other examples are efforts by federal agencies to effectively make equity planning and civil rights impact analyses core elements of the operation of federally assisted entities (Edson 2004; Johnson 2014; Yan 2013).

Concluding Thoughts

It is possible to think of Title VI as a holdover from a bygone era, when the pressing focus was on ending intentional discrimination by race. But that would be wrong. Title VI is far broader in its scope, the result of an early decision to interpret its reach liberally, followed by decades of private enforcement and, increasingly, more meaningful efforts on the part of the federal government itself, pressed into action by the end of private enforcement rights and the unceasing efforts of advocates and civil rights scholars. Today, it is expected that with participation in federal programs will come principles of non-discrimination in practice, embedded as a condition of program participation. In this regard, over its life, Title VI has emerged as an essential policy lever in the quest to bring fairness and equity to federally assisted programs. To be sure, much work remains, whether in mass transit, public housing, health care, education, parks and recreation, or other life endeavors that touch on the health and well-being of society. Although specific racial quotas are not possible, standards of fair treatment and equity-conscious planning are.

Two questions emerge from this analysis. The first is whether Title VI should be strengthened in the area of disparate impact enforcement. The second is what that strengthening might look like.

To answer the first question, one must ask whether it is still worthwhile to define certain problems in terms of race or national origin. Would we be better off focusing on economic inequality as the root cause of health inequity and moving away from a race discrimination framework instead, given the emotional fallout that can arise when one defines problems in terms of race? Put in the vernacular, with legal segregation behind us, is the juice not worth the squeeze in the case of Title VI?

The answer to the question of whether it is still important to use federal funding as a lever for achieving greater equity on racial grounds must be yes. To be sure, intentional, legal segregation has disappeared from the scene of publicly funded programs and services. But as long as policies produce racially identifiable results, it is vital to a nation with a racial history such as ours that the racial questions get asked even when income inequality plays a powerful role. This can most clearly be seen in the national dialogue that ensued in the wake of studies showing racially distinct outcomes in health care even when controlling for income and health status.

The power of knowing that race matters when formulating and enforcing policy in federally assisted programs is vividly evident in the tragedy of police-involved shootings in minority communities. It is Title VI that, in great part, has provided the legal leverage for the oversight of community policing policies and for altering the practices of police departments. Indeed, what made the Dallas 2016 police shooting especially painful was the fact that Dallas was recognized for the degree to which, over two generations, policing practices had been transformed. Title VI offers a policy lever over the vast array of policies that affect community health, because it travels wherever federal funding flows. The fact that police departments are subject to ongoing oversight may help the nation weather such terrible crises. In the current climate, we need a law that focuses on racial justice, because the nation still focuses on race, because people who are members of historically disadvantaged racial and ethnic minority groups continue to disproportionately feel the adverse effects of social and economic policy choices, and because what was true over fifty years ago is true today: public and private entities that accept public funding should be expected not merely to not discriminate on the basis of race but also to be actively involved in adapting programs and services in ways that achieve greater equity.

The second question is how, if Title VI remains powerful and relevant, its implementation might change to enable the law to better achieve its goals. One step would be to restore the private right of action to challenge practices and policies that are facially neutral but appear to have a racially measurable disproportionate impact. In the wake of the election of Donald Trump as president and the capture of both houses of Congress by Republicans, such a solution to the *Sandoval* problem is probably unlikely in the extreme. Of course, it is possible that judicial doctrine will evolve on its own, and that the United States Supreme Court will do an about-face on the question of whether private enforcement rights must be explicitly stated in law. This shift in jurisprudence is undoubtedly equally unlikely, particularly if a Republican president and Congress shift the Court further to the right. Thus, the use of Title VI by private parties in a judicial enforcement context is now precluded, at least where the problem of *de facto* discrimination is concerned; all eyes, instead, turn to government enforcement.

Here, even in a Trump administration, one might expect civil rights advocates to remain vigilant, placing administrative complaints before the federal agencies and the United States Justice Department on a range of issues. How rapidly and thoroughly these complaints will be acted on cannot be known, but the process of administrative advocacy remains very much alive. What probably will suffer in the coming years is the existence of a strong, government-initiated civil rights enforcement effort within the administration itself. As this article makes clear, even in times more conducive to framing issues as a civil rights matter, the executive branch has been relatively lethargic in its response to problems, with limited system monitoring and limited individual enforcement actions. Congress has been a significant part of this problem, refusing to fund civil rights enforcement in reasonable amounts.

Title VI enforcement agencies need budgets to collect data and commission research and analysis. They need staff. And they need to be an integral part of policy and programmatic development, not a mere commenter on regulations that already have been drafted. Title VI enforcement is not an add-on to federal program rules; it is part of the DNA of federal social programs. Just as a state housing agency does not qualify for federal funding if it fails to follow proper accounting practices, the agency loses its eligibility for federal assistance if its policies and practices violate the terms of Title VI and other fair housing laws.

In recent years the Obama administration, as noted, has made civil rights-related planning and resource allocation decisions a core element of its program oversight efforts. Expanding on these efforts means increasing the resources available for civil rights enforcement so that agencies can commission the empirical research studies needed to develop policies of general applicability that regulate grantee conduct, funding to collect the data needed to ensure compliance and test the effectiveness of policies in reducing disparate outcomes, and, of course, funding to properly investigate and enforce such policies when potential violations are reported. It is not enough for an agency to ask that a recipient sign a general Title VI compliance agreement and then simply reflect on what types of conduct and practices merit further investigation. As with the language access policies, recipients of federal funding need general directives and operating rules and the certainty of knowing that, if they comply with such rules, they will not be subject to further investigation. To function properly, civil rights compliance needs to be simply part of the process of policy development and program oversight. The Obama administration has taken steps in this direction, but it seems unlikely that the Trump administration will continue these practices. Indeed, early signals—from calls for retrenchment in public insurance financing under the Affordable Care Act to proposals that seek to dismantle public education rather than invest in it—are not promising, to put it mildly.

For this reason, research remains crucial. The research enterprise, if anything, grows more critical when government investment in civil rights enforcement wanes. Of particular importance is research that does not simply document racial and ethnic differences in access, quality, and outcomes, but that attempts to shed light on factors that may underlie problems, even when those factors involve asking uncomfortable questions. When researching disparities, it is valuable to examine patient preference, community culture, and individual value and belief systems. But it is equally important—and undoubtedly harder—to ask institutions questions about their own preferences, their own culture, and their own value and belief systems, as embodied in their policies and practices.

But there is a paradox here. Research designed to get at the policy underpinnings of disparities patterns is closely associated with enforcement. This means that not only is such work costly, complex, and time consuming, but it is also the result of direct funding by government agencies that seek answers in a civil rights context in order to better understand the potential for discriminatory effects that may result from the implementation of federal programs and policies. This type of deeper research can be expected to wither in an era of government disfavor of civil rights enforcement. In this case, the role of private funders—and of agencies and institutions that themselves that seek to more clearly understand the impact of their own policies and practices on the people and communities they serve—becomes paramount.

▪ ▪ ▪

Sara Rosenbaum is the Harold and Jane Hirsh professor and founding chair, Department of Health Policy, Milken Institute School of Public Health, George Washington University. She has provided public service to six presidential administrations and twenty-one Congresses, and is known for her work on the expansion of Medicaid, the expansion of community health centers, patients' rights in managed care, civil rights and health care, and national health reform. She is the lead author of *Law and the American Health Care System*, 2nd ed. (Foundation Press, 2012), a landmark textbook that explores in depth the interaction of American law and the US health care system.
sarar@gwu.edu

Sara Schmucker is a senior research associate in the Department of Health Policy and Management at the Milken Institute School of Public Health, George Washington University. She received her Juris Doctor degree from the George Washington University School of Law.

References

Abernathy, Charles F. 1981. "Title VI and the Constitution: A Regulatory Model for Defining 'Discrimination.'" *Georgetown Law Journal* 70, no. 1: 1–49.

Abernathy, Charles F. 2006. *Civil Rights and Constitutional Litigation: Cases and Materials.* St. Paul, MN: Thomson/West.

Byrd, W. Michael, and Linda A. Clayton. 2001. "Race, Medicine, and Health Care in the United States: A Historical Survey." *Journal of the National Medical Association* 93, no. 3 suppl.: 11S–34S.

Edson, Scott Michael. 2004. "Title VI or Bust? A Practical Evaluation of Title VI of the 1964 Civil Rights Act As an Environmental Justice Remedy." *Fordham Environmental Law Review* 16, no. 1: 141–79.

Harvard Law Review Association. 2001. "Leading Cases; B. Civil Rights Act," *Harvard Law Review* 115: 497.

Johnson, Olatunde C. A. 2014. "Lawyering That Has No Name: Title VI and the Meaning of Private Enforcement." *Stanford Law Review* 66, no. 6: 1293–1332.

Mank, Bradford. 2007. "Title VI and the Warren County Protests." *Golden Gate University Environmental Law Journal* 1, no. 1: 73–89.

Perez, Thomas E. 2002. "The Civil Rights Dimension of Racial and Ethnic Disparities in Health Status." In *Unequal Treatment: Confronting Racial and Ethnic Disparities in Health Care*, edited by Brian D. Smedley, Adrienne Y. Stith, and Alan R. Nelson, 626-63. Washington, DC: Institute of Medicine (US) Committee on Understanding and Eliminating Racial and Ethnic Disparities in Health Care.

Purdum, Todd S. 2014. *An Idea Whose Time Has Come: Two Presidents, Two Parties, and the Battle for the Civil Rights Act of 1964.* New York: Henry Holt and Company.

Rosenbaum, Sara, and David M. Frankford. 2012. *Law and the American Health Care System.* New York: Foundation.

Rosenbaum, Sara, and Joel Teitelbaum. 2003. "Civil Rights Enforcement in the Modern Healthcare System: Reinvigorating the Role of the Federal Government in the Aftermath of *Alexander v. Sandoval.*" *Yale Journal of Health Policy, Law and Ethics* 3, no. 2: 215–52.

Rubin-Wills, Jessica. 2012. "Language Access Advocacy after *Sandoval*: A Case Study of Administrative Enforcement outside the Shadow of Judicial Review." *New York University Review of Law and Social Change* 36, no. 3: 465–511.

Schulman, Kevin A., Jesse A. Berlin, William Harless, Jon F. Kerner, Shyrl Sistrunk, Bernard J. Gersh, Ross Dubé et al. 1999. "The Effect of Race and Sex on Physicians' Recommendations for Cardiac Catheterization." *New England Journal of Medicine* 340: 618–26.

Smith, David Barton. 1999. *Health Care Divided: Race and Healing a Nation.* Ann Arbor: University of Michigan Press.

Steege, Sarah G. 2011. "Finding a Cure in the Courts: A Private Right of Action for Disparate Impact in Health Care." *Michigan Journal of Race and Law* 16, no. 2: 439–67.

Watson, Sidney D. 1990. "Reinvigorating Title VI: Defending Health Care Discrimination— It Shouldn't Be So Easy." *Fordham Law Review* 58, no. 5: 939–78.

Williams, David R., and Pamela Braboy Jackson. 2005. "Social Sources of Racial Disparities in Health." *Health Affairs* 24, no. 2: 325–34.

Yan, Jerett. 2013. "Rousing the Sleeping Giant: Administrative Enforcement of Title VI and New Routes to Equity in Transit Planning." *California Law Review* 101, no. 4: 1131–80.

Cancer and Race: What They Tell Us about the Emerging Focus of Health Equity

Keith Wailoo
Princeton University

Abstract This article examines the history of concepts and frames (such as "equity" or "disparities") and how these frames have guided public policies and explanations about differences in health across the population. Considering the emblematic case of cancer, which has stimulated long and heated debate over social, economic, and biological causes, the article argues that the vocabularies of health reform are both semantic and also deeply political—framing different reform agendas. The article describes the evolving US debate over the biological, social, or environmental origins of differential cancer mortality along lines of social difference and race, tracing important shifts and reversal over time. Through this analysis, the article explains how and why equity concerns have figured (sometimes implicitly, sometimes explicitly) in health reform discussions, often in tension with other frames. It examines how Americans have used these frameworks to justify different kinds of action and inaction, concluding with a discussion of how these frameworks of "disparities" and "equity" should be understood today in scientific, political, and policy discourse.[1]

Keywords race, health equity, cancer, health disparities

Recently, the focus of many reform-minded scholars, funders, and some policy makers has shifted from disparities—reducing inequalities in mortality, incidence, and survival across groups—to equity, defined as focusing on "those disparities that can be traced to unequal, systemic, economic, and social conditions" (McNeill Ransom et al. 2011: 94). The shift in terminology is not merely semantic, but represents (at its heart) a

---

1. This reflection essay draws heavily on my book, *How Cancer Crossed the Color Line* (Oxford University Press, 2010).

Journal of Health Politics, Policy and Law, Vol. 42, No. 5, October 2017
DOI 10.1215/03616878-3940441   © 2017 by Duke University Press

new programmatic vision—it aims to focus on unjust structural conditions that shape health outcomes. In other words, while disparities (in health outcomes) might have many roots, from social class to biology and environment, the focus on inequities seeks to call attention to differences that are created by malleable social circumstances.

There is both a rhetorical and political strategy at the heart of this shift in language—narrowing the scope and target of reform while honing in on the health effects linked to social status and environment. Equity-focused scholars and reformers ask, why should zip code and the social circumstances of one's birth, upbringing, and life make such a difference in health outcomes? Championing this new approach, for example, the Robert Wood Johnson Foundation has insisted that many disparities in health are rooted in disparities in structural opportunity. "When it comes to health across cities," commented Catherine Malone and Dwayne Proctor, "zip codes are unequal and so are health outcomes. . . . Our goal is greater health equity in America." According to this ideal, if health equity is achieved, "the end result should be decreased health disparities."[2] Embracing this new call to action, as one reform-minded group of scholars have put it: "The goal of health equity will not immediately eliminate all health disparities, but [it] will provide a foundation for moving closer to that goal" (Health Equity).[3]

As policy frames, terms like "equity" and "disparities" are calls to action—highlighting achievable goals. Since at least the early 1970s, for example, reducing cancer disparities has focused epidemiologists, public health officials, scholars, and others on expanding cancer screening, ensuring access to prompt diagnosis and treatment, and evening out chances of survival. The inequalities are stark. Black women with lower incidence of breast cancer than white women were experiencing higher mortality, why? Such disparities in cancer incidence, mortality, and survival had their origins in differential access to care, reformers argued. Narrowing the gap became the crucial measure of progress. But skeptics promoted another contention—that some disparities could be rooted in differences in biology and genetic risk—and, as such, were not as easily "fixed" or

2. Catherine Malone and Dwayne Proctor, "Shaking Up Systems to Achieve Health Equity," (May 17, 2016). www.rwjf.org/en/culture-of-health/2016/03/shaking-up-systems.html.

3. The idea of equity has attracted increasing interest—coming into wider use among health scholars and reformers over the past decade or so, and framing an old challenge (the problem of addressing population-wide health inequalities and disparities) from a new perspective—not by trying to lower the gaps in mortality between groups but by looking at each group and attempting to achieve the highest level of health possible, bearing in mind different socioeconomic conditions. Where disparities research focused on reducing differences in outcomes, the new focus on inequities focuses on a related, yet distinct, problem—fixing avoidable or unjust differences in health.

remedied. Unlike those health disparities rooted in social and economic inequalities, some disparities might never go away, they contended. For the last few decades, this biological claim has deviled those who seek to reduce cancer disparities. The inequity argument can be seen as a new chapter in this ongoing debate, sidestepping the biology question by refocusing not on striving for equality but for equal opportunity and on injustice.[4]

Tensions in the vocabulary of health reform (equity, disparities, socio-economic roots, genetic, and so on) have guided public policy interventions for decades. In what follows, I consider the history of how cancer differences have been framed—an emblematic case of how frameworks have mattered in policy and society. To look at cancer is to see shifts and tensions in the unfolding debate over the origins of differential health. The recent focus on "equity" is merely the latest chapter in this century-long debate. Yet, the focus on equity is not fundamentally new; the concept, even if not the word itself, has often figured in health reform and justified different kinds of political reform.

Framing of Cancer and Difference: Before Disparities

Before Americans began focusing on cancer disparities in the 1960s and 1970s, how did they frame inequalities in mortality across the population? One hundred years ago, most health experts believed that health disparities were natural—part of a normal fabric of the social and biological order. Few experts would have championed a cause or call to reduce cancer disparities because any disparities were seen as defined by different bodies and different biological risks. It was, for example, a disease associated simultaneously with longevity, biology, and social circumstances. The longer you lived and the more you were able to avoid mortality from the dominant infectious diseases of the time (such as tuberculosis), the more

---

4. In 2016, for example, when the Susan G. Komen Foundation announced a new $27 million "health equity" initiative to reduce breast cancer deaths in African American communities, they threw their weight behind the idea that it was not biology but "local programs like screening, treatment assistance, emergency financial aid, medical supplies, and living expenses" that determined death and survival. "Susan G. Komen Announces $27 Million Health Equity Initiative to Reduce Breast Cancer Deaths in African-American Community—10-City Initiative Complements Komen's Decades-long Service to Medically Underserved," "African American women are almost 40 percent more likely to die of breast cancer than white women in the U.S. and in some cities, that number is as high as 74 percent. That makes this a public health crisis that must be addressed immediately," said Komen President and CEO Dr. Judith A. Salerno. "We are deeply appreciative of friends and partners who are working with us to do so." ww5.komen.org/News /Susan-G--Komen-Announces-$27-Million-Health-Equity-Initiative-To-Reduce-Breast-Cancer -Deaths-In-African-American-Community.html.

likely you (and your social group) were to die from cancer. Tuberculosis was a disease of the underprivileged; cancer was a disease of the longer lived and well-to-do.

Racial biology, so called, also figured prominently in this framing of mortality differences with white people seen as carrying higher risks. "Without exception," wrote the influential Prudential Life Insurance company statistician, Frederick Hoffman, "the general cancer mortality is higher for the white population than the Negro" (Hoffman 1915). Racial behavior, in experts' view, also explained differential rates of venereal disease, tuberculosis, and infectious disease. Hoffman and many other health experts saw these differences as outgrowths of natural differences in the way white and black Americans lived. For experts, these differences in lifestyle and social circumstances were not biological, but largely social.

Experts of this era framed cancer as a disease of civilization, and saw "primitive" societies as relatively protected from its ravages. So too did class differences frame the cancer question. In an era where infectious diseases (tuberculosis, pneumonia, and others) were the leading cause of mortality, poor people lived in worlds where infectious disease, childhood mortality, and early death dominated. By contrast, better-off people who enjoyed longer life spans survived these threats in greater numbers. The consequence of their survival was that they lived long enough to reach the so-called "cancer age"—a dominant view that linked cancer to privilege, aging, and higher social status. If cancer was a disease of privilege, then the absence of cancer in lower-class groups was a point of curiosity for experts. Writing in his book *Cancer: Its Origins, Its Development, and Its Self-Perpetuation*, New York surgeon Willy Meyer wrote that "primitive people . . . in the familiar character of their restful surroundings, would almost seem to be on a par with the fish of the ocean, the life of which is spent in place indifference in the never-changing salt solution and its always equal temperature" (Meyer, 1931: 236). For such experts, cancer disparities were embedded in the different cultures and ways of life of blacks and whites.

In the first half of the century, however, a handful of shrewd dissenters ignored this civilization-primitivism framework, and understood that cancer mortality differences were themselves the product of a society with unequal access to resources. For them, different social factors explained disparate outcomes. As one expert wrote in the *American Journal of Cancer* in 1935, "Cancer appears to be less prevalent in the colored population," but statistics were notoriously unreliable. "Undoubtedly, differences in diagnostic practice [that is, in access to diagnosis] have some effect upon our statistics on cancer death rates" (Holmes 1935). In this view, well-to-do people only appeared to have higher cancer rates because they had greater access to diagnostic services and care. For Louis Dublin, insurance access (life insurance) confounded what was known and unknown about cancer. As chief statistician at Metropolitan Life Insurance, he understood that differences in insurance coverage (not only in access to diagnosis) skewed the cancer mortality data—shaping theories about who had cancer and where cancer resided in society. As Dublin wrote in 1928, if there was one serious limitation in the cancer mortality data, it was that "the business is conducted, very largely in the urban areas. . . . The conditions which prevail in the rural South, where a large proportion of the Negroes live, are therefore not closely reflected by the insurance experience" (Dublin 1928). A new idea took root here—the notion that access to health care services influenced the cancer statistics and the mortality trends.

Dublin's insights were not driven by a concern with equity; rather, his words illustrate a growing sensitivity to the fact that existing frames of primitivism and civilization were inadequate, and did not explain differential cancer mortality. For such observers, the old framework was misguided and deceptive. Nor did the old frame offer a plan of action. Structural questions such as unequal access explained why some died from cancer and others did not. For these critical observers, new frameworks were needed to explain the social origins of these disease differences.

Social Inequities and Health—the Rise of a Modern Frame

New times called for new frameworks. In the context of the Great Depression and the New Deal (and the growing pressure on government to collect evidence and to respond to widespread economic deprivation), the 1930s and 1940s witnessed a more explicit reform focus on the social origins of health outcomes. Expanding New Deal government brought more robust federal and state involvement in reducing the toll of infectious disease mortality and childhood mortality, and reshaped how US society began to grapple with cancer. Programs such as the National Cancer Institute, the US Public Health Service, and Social Security were created as efforts to enhance access, and to reduce inequities across groups. The social welfare agenda of New Deal reform was sweeping, even if at the same time these programs existed within (and continued to promote) a segregated racial society.

Mid-twentieth-century social and economic forces were gradually altering awareness of cancer disparities—shifting not only the idea that cancer was a disease of privilege, but also establishing new views about the social origins of cancer. For example, the migration of black Americans into cities where cancer diagnosis was more common meant an increasing likelihood of diagnosis, albeit in struggling public hospitals and not in white-only or segregated facilities. In the context of migration, old regional differences in access to care were accompanied, and in a way displaced, by new institutional ones. Diagnosis was slowly improving everywhere, but not evenly. But also government programs played a role, as the US Public Health Service initiated new programs such as the Ten Cities Cancer Surveys, pushing government statisticians like Harold Dorn to look at cancer statistics with new eyes. All these trends—in migration, diagnostic science, and government—slowly eradicated the old primitivism-civilization framework of cancer.

At mid-century, health was in epidemiological transition in America, and most experts acknowledged that disparities were never static but always evolving. With infectious disease in decline as a major cause of mortality, the death toll from chronic degenerative diseases like cancer rose to take their place. As old disease divisions disappeared, new ones appeared—giving rise to a new face of health differences during the period from 1940 through the 1960s. More and more, cancer was understood as an "equal opportunity disease," and one that should—in the natural course of things—affect each group equally. To the extent that outcomes differed, experts began to ask why. And it is here (in this society where infectious disease mortality fell across the board, if unevenly) that a modern focus on cancer disparities emerged. And by the 1960s and 1970s, in the context of a rising focus on civil rights and health care reform, the fight against those disparities began to take shape.

Adding further complexity to this epidemiological picture, cancer itself was changing as a result of medical and scientific specialization—the malady no longer being regarded by experts as one singular disease, but as coming in many different types, each of which told a different story about disparities across the population and methods of prevention. In some cancers, behavior (not race or biology per se) seemed to be a major factor when discussing disparities. As one 1950 Congressional Report on the new cancer trends highlighted, breast cancer rates in the US population told the story of higher incidence among whites as compared to nonwhites. Experts theorized that these disparities could be explained by social factors (difference in behaviors such as rates of breastfeeding). Lung cancer, on the other hand, revealed higher incidence in whites than in nonwhites; but here, studies suggest another social factor (cigarette smoking) played a dominant role in the rising incidence and mortality among white men. By contrast, cervical cancer showed higher incidence among nonwhites, provoking some experts to wonder about the role of sexual behaviors. By the 1950s, then, many observers had developed a behaviorist framework to explain these disparities—theorizing that cancer differences were rooted not in biology, as once believed, or in civilization, but in social differences in increasingly stigmatized behaviors. To fix these disparities, it was said, one needed to address the underlying behaviors—smoking, sex, and practices associated with maternity.

By the years after World War II, a new face of cancer inequality had arisen—one that was far more complicated and confusing than the prewar picture, and one where an active debate about multiple causes and different methods of intervention and prevention had arisen. Disparities came in many shades. By the 1950s, even as some experts linked cervical cancer to behavior, for example, new diagnostic tests like the Pap smear—linking early diagnosis to increased survival—meant that differences in access to diagnosis figured more than ever in mortality differences. With expanding access to testing, such cancers became more clinically and socially visible at earlier stages of development. Yet, it would take another decade before experts would frame these differences in access as questions of equity and social injustice.

The 1960s health care debates over Medicare and Medicaid provoked a quantum shift of framework by squarely associating health outcomes with differences in access to health services, and identified health insurance as the crucial factor separating the haves from the have-nots in society. The World War II environment had seen this new framework slowly unfold, with Americans witnessing the rising cost of health care and the expansion of private health insurance—a set of developments that left behind many in the population (particularly the elderly and poor). Since the 1930s, out-of-pocket payments for health care expenditures had risen steadily, driven by a greater number of tests and therapies. By the late 1940s, private insurers had entered the market (covering growing numbers of Americans, often through their employers), and ensuring access to an expanding market of high-cost goods. Systematically, these trends created the growing gap between those with and without private health insurance. This new political reality explains much about what drove President Truman and other Democrats to push for national health insurance in the late 1940s, it underpinned the establishment of disability provisions in Social Security in the 1950s under Eisenhower, and it defined the pressures building into the early 1960s to pass Medicare and Medicaid. The central reform ideal of this era became expanding access to those who were most vulnerable, including the disabled, the elderly, and the poor, and to even the playing field in the name of fairness and equity.

Although the term *equity* was not widely used at the time in these debates, a powerful equity-based framework defined these political battles. The unfairness of the emerging health insurance gap was palpable. "Almost everyone realizes that a great mass of the old people do not have the savings, and cannot depend upon their children, to pay for the doctors, hospitals, nursing homes, and drugs which, because they are aging, they need more than do younger people," wrote Walter Lippman in 1960.[5] This insurance gap opened a vexing new stage in the American debate—hinging not on whether there were inequities in the emerging health care system, but what to do about such inequalities and injustices.

In the years leading up to the passage of Medicare and Medicaid in 1965 (and coinciding with the peak of civil rights legislation), the inherent unfairness of the US health care system circumscribed every discussion about health and society in America. It was widely assumed that structural injustice led to disparate health outcomes—cutting along lines of race, class, and age. This insistence fueled programmatic innovations in government and social services, and spurred a decades-long debate that carries over into our own era. Today's framework for thinking about equity owes much to this era of activism and political reform. Yet, this earlier era also produced something else in its wake: a new "disparities" framework focusing on reducing epidemiological gaps and seeking equality in disease outcomes (such as cancer) across groups.

The Discovery of Racial Health Disparities

The passage of Medicare drew millions of elderly Americans into what Louis Dublin had called the "insurance experience," and thus also into the medical care system and, as a consequence, provided more comparable access across lines of class and race to the elderly (Dublin 1928). Yet, new gaps in health experience across the population began to appear even as old gaps persisted. With expanding access through private and public insurance, for example, the data on cancer incidence and mortality began to shift. Seven years after Medicare's passage, health statisticians marveled at

5. Walter Lippman, "Medical Care for the Aged," *New York Herald Tribune*, June 16, 1960, 20.

an apparent inversion of the old theory of race and cancer. Where early twentieth-century experts had labeled cancer as a white disease, new studies in the early 1970s observed that cancer "was not just a white disease" anymore (Slater 1979). As *Newsweek* reported the findings of an influential Howard University study:

> The death rate from cancer in the U.S. has been rising steadily since the beginning of the century, due in part to the control of such major killers as tuberculosis and pneumonia. But recently, epidemiologists have discerned a striking new feature of this trend . . . a sudden, sharp rise in cancer deaths among Negroes. ("Cancer in Negroes," 1979)

The Howard study observed that, from 1950 to 1967, mortality had risen from 147 per 100,000 to 177 per 100,000 for African Americans while the rate had stabilized at 150 for whites. Epidemiologists, cancer specialists, and society at large had discovered a new face of cancer disparities. Cancer had mysteriously crossed the color line. Narrowing this worrisome gap became an epidemiological and a political concern.

The early 1970s marked the beginning of a decades-long focus on racial health disparities—with the explicit aim of determining why the gap had grown—and attempting to reduce those gaps. The National Cancer Institute created a new SEER program (Surveillance, Epidemiology, and End-Results) to track these inequalities along multiple axes: cancer diagnosis, treatment, outcomes, and survival. Over the next four decades, the drive for reduced health inequalities seemed only common sense—especially given the recent discovery of the "alarming increase" in cancer deaths and the vital need to reverse these historical trends. For the next generation in this post–Civil Rights/post-Medicare era, few, if any, spoke of health inequities; the new watchword, the potent framework for reform, was attacking "disparities."

But the "disparities" focus also invited, by the 1980s, a skeptical response—the contention that disparities in population health had many origins, and that resolving them by aiming for equivalence in health outcomes across groups was too ambitious. The agenda of health equality ignored the complex social, biological, behavioral, dietary, and economic origins of disease differences across the population. Skepticism took both epidemiological and political form. If the dream of health equality rested on the liberal, reform-oriented idea that an activist government could address these challenges, this insistence gave way to conservative skepticism in the late 1970s and 1980s. "In this present crisis, government," President Ronald Reagan announced in his 1981 inaugural address, "is not the solution to our problem. Government *is* the problem" (Reagan 1981). With the rise of a less active federal government and with the declining commitment to 1960s civil rights agendas (and as the US political climate became more conservative and wary of government activism), the focus on health care injustice waned—and the commitment to addressing disparities faced powerful headwinds. At the same time, a new scientific skepticism appeared—the growing conceit that genetic and biological differences might explain some cancer disparities. An old biological fatalism (akin with the early twentieth century's primitivism-civilization framework) had reemerged. This genetic perspective resonated with the political climate—both cautioning against liberal intervention and the pursuit of equality.

Into the 1990s, a generation of research had documented the many competing frameworks on health disparities. Looking back across the century, we must understand these contentious frameworks—whether cancer was a social and economic disease, a genetic disease, an environmental ailment, a behavioral malady, or a disease caused by diet, etc.—as a debate in which science remained deeply intertwined with an unfolding political and reform discussion. In light of this enduring competition to control the debate over cancer, the "disparities" framework called attention to the programmatic pursuit of equality even if, by the 1990s, the complexity of that agenda had become clear. The new focus on "inequity" (a term often referring to unfair and avoidable differences linked to injustices such as corruption, exclusion, or governance practices) should be understood in this historical context. In the still-unfolding debate over cancer and health differences, a new focus on inequities shifts us away from the pursuit of equality and away from the biological discussion, and points us toward identifying and addressing the underlying social or structural injustices known to be driving those inequalities. In 1999, for example, the Institute of Medicine drew attention to the "unequal burden of cancer"—noting one example of inequity hidden within cancer disparities: African Americans have lower breast cancer incidence than their white peers (suggesting lower biological risk), yet they have higher mortality and lower survival chance compared to whites (Haynes and Smedley 1999). In the intervening two decades, not much has changed in this epidemiological picture. Examples like these in the cancer world (and in other realms of health) illustrate why and how a new equity-based framework emerged, focusing not on disparities alone but also on injustice, and thereby aiming to restart a stalled political reform agenda.

Framing Health through Equity and Equality

The recent scholarly or reform focus on health equity is thus not fundamentally new, but it represents a kind of circling back to older strategies along the long and winding road of health reform. Bearing in mind the long history of cancer, civilization, behavior, migration, social status, and race, what can we conclude about these shifting vocabularies of health and the rise of a new language of equity?

The focus on equity is a refinement of the previous generation's focus on the pursuit of inequality, a pursuit that has been frustrated and (to some extent) unsuccessful. In retrospect, we can see the quest for *equality* in cancer outcomes as born from a specific time when the shocking, recent 1960s divergence captured public health attention and cried out for a reversal. Today, some fifty years later, the ideal of achieving health equality across all groups seems unreasonable—especially as we acknowledge just how many complex social, behavioral, biological, and economic factors shape disparate outcomes across groups, and as the drive to achieve health equality has been frustrated by political and biological skepticism.

The focus on health equity turns our attention away from equality per se, avoids the critique leveled at those who aimed toward health equality, and avoids the familiar biological criticisms—pointing instead toward addressing fundamental issues where health differences have demonstrable origins in social justice and fairness. As the history of American cancer discourse highlights, there have always been fierce competing frameworks for characterizing health differences across the population—debates that are at once scientific and political. The call for health equity is the latest chapter in this unfolding drama. It originates in a frustrating space—with an acknowledgment that reducing "disparities" one disease at a time has been a difficult road. It also originates with a powerful hope—that a new agenda focused on addressing those social differences that clearly and demonstrably produce disease differences can bring progress in a challenging and ever-changing political climate. Every framework, of course, has its limits—telling only part of the story of health and health reform. Disparities, in many ways, is the language of striving for epidemiological equivalence and bringing mortality and morbidity statistics into rough alignment; but the idea of closing the gap was, by definition, both grand yet frustrating and limited. By contrast, the striving for health equity injects the language of social justice into the health debate. The pursuit of *equity*, however, has this limitation—it focuses on a goal that is extremely difficult to measure. Looking ahead then, should the goal of cancer reform be reducing disparities or equity? Clearly, the answer must be not a commitment to one or the other, but to both continuing on the road to reducing disparities and developing measures and a science to support the pursuit of health equity.

* * *

Keith Wailoo is Townsend Martin professor of history and public affairs at Princeton University, where he is appointed in History and the Woodrow Wilson School of Public and International Affairs. His books include *Pain: A Political History, How Cancer Crossed the Color Line,* and *Dying in the City of the Blues: Sickle Cell Anemia and the Politics of Race and Health.* His edited volumes include *Medicare and Medicaid at Fifty: America's Entitlements in the Age of Affordable Care.* Other writings have appeared in *Lancet, Bulletin of the History of Medicine, New York Times, Daily Beast,* and *New England Journal of Medicine.*
kwailoo@princeton.edu

References

"Cancer in Negroes." 1972. *Newsweek.* May 29, 77.

Dublin, Louis. 1928. "The Health of the Negro," *Annals of the American Academy of Political and Social Science* 140 (November): 77–85. Later revised and updated in Louis Dublin, "The Problem of Negro Health as Revealed by Vital Statistics," *Journal of Negro Education* 6 (July 1937): 268–75.

Haynes, M. A., and B. D. Smedley, eds. 1999. *The Unequal Burden of Cancer: An Assessment of NIH Research and Programs for Ethnic Minorities and the Medically Underserved.* Washington, DC: National Academy.

Health EquityInstitute for Research, Practice, and Policy. n.d. San Francisco State University. https://healthequity.sfsu.edu/content/defining-health-equity (accessed June 11, 2017).

Hoffman, Frederick. 1915. Quoted in Helen Kirchoff and R. H. Rigdon. "Frequency of Cancer in the White and Negro: A Study Based Upon Necropsies." *Southern Medical Journal* 49 (August 1956): 834.

Holmes, Samuel Jackson. "The Differential Mortality from Cancer in the White and Colored Population." *American Journal of Cancer* 25 (October 1935): 358–76.

Lippman, Walter. 1960. "Medical Care for the Aged." *New York Herald Tribune,* June 16.

Malone, Catherine, and Dwayne Proctor. 2016. "Shaking Up Systems to Achieve Health Equity." May 17. www.rwjf.org/en/culture-of-health/2016/03/shaking-up -systems.html.

McNeill Ransom, Montrece, Amelia Greiner, Chris Kochtitzky, and Kristin S. Major. 2011. "Pursuing Health Equity: Zoning Codes and Public Health." *Journal of Law, Medicine, and Ethics* 39 Suppl 1: S94–S97.

Meyer, Willy. 1931. *Cancer: Its Origins, Its Development, and Its Self-Perpetuation.* New York: Paul Hoeber.

Reagan, Ronald. "Inaugural Address, January 20, 1981," The American Presidency Project. www.presidency.ucsb.edu/ws/?pid=43130.

Slater, Jack. 1979. "The Terrible Rise of Cancer Among Blacks." *Ebony* (November): 131.

"Susan G. Komen Announces $27 Million Health Equity Initiative to Reduce Breast Cancer Deaths in African-American Women." 2016. September 14. ww5.komen .org/News/Susan-G--Komen-Announces-$27-Million-Health-Equity-Initiative-To -Reduce-Breast-Cancer-Deaths-In-African-American-Community.html.

Framing Health Equity: US Health Disparities in Comparative Perspective

Julia F. Lynch
Isabel M. Perera
University of Pennsylvania

Abstract In this article we explore systematically the different conceptions of health equity in key national health policy documents in the United States, the United Kingdom, and France. We find substantial differences across the three countries in the characterization of group differences (by SES, race/ethnicity, or territory), and the theorized causes of health inequalities (socioeconomic structures versus health care system features). In all three countries, reports throughout the period alluded at least minimally to inequalities in social determinants as the underlying cause of health inequalities. However, even in the reports with the strongest attachment to this causal model, the authors stop well short of advocating the redistribution of power and resources that would likely be necessary to redress these inequalities.

Keywords health inequality, framing, cross-national comparisons

Introduction

The health enjoyed by members of groups defined by economic, racial and ethnic, geographic, or gender differences, among others, can vary dramatically. Readers of this journal are well aware of some of the gaps in life mortality, morbidity, and access to health care between, for example, African Americans and white Americans, those living in rural and urban areas, or people with a college degree and those with less than high school education. Given this multiplicity of inequalities in health status and health care, how do governments choose to frame the issue of health equity, identify the underlying causes of inequalities in health, and craft appropriate policy responses? In this article we analyze major government

Journal of Health Politics, Policy and Law, Vol. 42, No. 5, October 2017
DOI 10.1215/03616878-3940450 © 2017 by Duke University Press

reports from the United States, the United Kingdom, and France over the last thirty years to identify common trends and differences in these governments' approaches to health equity. Comparative analysis reminds us that the approach taken in any one setting is not an inevitable outgrowth of the fact of group differences in health. Instead, how governments frame health equity as a problem for politics, and the policies they advance to try to address that problem, are contingent. While the weight of history, institutions, and political cultures may tip the balance toward one framing or another, political communities can and do make choices about what to do in the face of inequities in health. The present analysis strives to clarify the choices that we have already made, and to offer, through comparative analysis of countries that are similar to ours, a broader vision of what might be possible in the future.

Policy elites at the international level and in European countries often use the term *health inequalities* more or less interchangeably with health inequities. The European Union, for example, defines health inequalities as "preventable and unjust differences in health status or in the distribution of health determinants between different population groups." Similarly, in French policy discourse, the term "social" in the apparently neutral phrase *inégalités sociales de santé* (ISS) references health differences linked to socioeconomic position, which are generally regarded as unjust. In other words, in the discourse of European policy makers and researchers, the term *health inequality* has come to denote a policy problem (Bardach 1996) that has been identified as such at least partly because it is seen as inequitable. In the United States, by contrast, discussions of group differences in health more frequently use the term *disparity*, which in many instances does not include a fairness judgment.

Our findings suggest that the difference in language and framing does not simply reflect the fact that research communities in the United States and Europe have developed somewhat independently of each other. American and European policy communities conceptualize the problem of health inequalities differently, and in ways that are related to the causal models and policy solutions that are advanced in different countries to address health equity. However, we find that in all three countries, the policy recommendations that are espoused in government documents fall short of the remedies implied by understandings of the processes generating inequity in health. This suggests that reducing health inequalities may be even more politically difficult than researchers generally think; but it also shows that there is room for a reframing of health disparities in the United States to accommodate a broader scope of policy responses.

Background

In most of the international and cross-national research literature in epidemiology and public health, scholars measure or attempt to explain health inequalities that are related to differences in socioeconomic status (SES, usually operationalized as income, type of occupation, or educational attainment). In the international policy community, researchers and activists characterize health inequalities as preventable, unfair, and hence deserving of policy attention to the extent that they result from underlying social inequalities that are produced by our political, economic, and social systems (CSDH 2008; Whitehead 1991). Yet, differences in health status across social groups defined by characteristics other than SES— for example, by ethnicity or race; gender; disability status; or geography— could also be considered preventable and unjust, depending on the circumstances. So, while important policy documents produced by the World Health Organization (most recently, the 2008 report of WHO's Commission on the Social Determinants of Health, chaired by Englishman Sir Michael Marmot) frame health equity primarily in terms of SES, there is nothing "natural" or inevitable about this framing.

Consider how a recent report from the Centers for Disease Control (CDC Health 2015) presents infant mortality rates. Differences are listed by race and ethnicity (11.3 African American infant deaths per 1,000 births, compared to 5.1 white infant deaths; 5.1 for Hispanics, 8.1 for American Indian or Alaska Natives; and 4.2 for Asian or Pacific Islanders), and by state and territory (ranging from 11.1 in American Samoa to 4.2 in Massachusetts) (CDC Health 2015, table 12). Data on infant mortality by income level or occupational status are noticeably absent.

Of course, different forms of inequalities may overlap, and when we decide to disentangle them it entails choices that are ultimately conceptual and political, rather than merely technical. Take as an example the relationship between racial (black-white) and socioeconomic health inequalities in the United States. Because race and SES are correlated but not completely, it is possible to estimate the "effects" of race and SES on health separately using observational data. Scholars have debated whether this is a desirable practice, however. Williams (1999) argues that many traditional measures of SES have distinctly different effects on whites and African Americans, so that controlling for SES can "account for" much of the observed racial disparity in health status while substantially underplaying the role of institutional and individual forms of racism on health status. Reed and Chowkwanyun (2012) go one step further, demonstrating that the practice of identifying and measuring racial disparities in health is itself rooted in the development of American social science and policy research, where some of the more complex relationships between race and class have been buried under a dominant narrative about durable racial inequalities.

By framing inequalities as either "about" SES or "about" race or some other group, policy makers can simplify, or even perhaps obscure, the complexity of the overlapping boundaries between social groups that are defined in different ways. Policy frames involve a definition of the social problem, a causal story about where that problem comes from, and a policy prescription—each of which may invoke a moral evaluation that determines who is responsible for causing and/or treating the problem (Entman 1993; Stone 1989; Verloo 2005). How policy frames are constructed and employed therefore has implications for politics—who is to blame, who is responsible—and can be expected to shape the policies intended to address the problem.

We observe in this article that health equity frames vary across countries. A systematic, comparative analysis of how national policy elites frame differences in health status serves to denaturalize health inequities, and to make more easily visible some of the institutions, ideas, and interests that shape contemporary definitions of inequality. To our knowledge, only one other study adopts a comparative approach to the discursive construction of health equity that includes the United States (Docteur and Berenson 2014; for comparative work not involving the United States, see Lynch 2016; Vallgårda 2007[1]). Docteur and Berenson (2014) compare American health equity frames to those employed in European Union policy documents, but the EU in fact has little competence over the health and social policies of its member states. We instead compare the frames employed by authors of health policy documents in the United States and those that appear in documents produced by actors with the authority to affect public policies related to health in the UK and France. We conducted a systematic sampling of government documents—that is, documents produced by policy makers with the intention of shaping public policy—to examine these differences across the three cases.

Research Design and Methods

Frame Analysis of Government Reports. Discourses or conversations about policy problems, like discussions about anything else, are inherently

---

1. The Gusmano et al. 2010 comparative study of New York, Paris, and London is a useful guide to health policies that affect population health at the metropolitan level in the three countries we consider, but in that volume there is no attention to the alternative framings of health equity.

incomplete. Frames do their work by activating schema in the minds of recipients of messages, who then use these schema unconsciously to "fill in the blanks" between elements of a problem in order to construct responses that seem reasonable (van Gorp 2007). Within the arena of public health, policy frames can affect whether an issue gets on the agenda (Stone 1989), shape policy responses to a problem (e.g., Kenterelidou 2012; Saguy and Riley 2005), and affect public beliefs and attitudes about policy choices, including policies related to health inequalities (e.g., Gollust and Lynch 2011; Lynch and Gollust 2010; Rigby et al. 2009).

Tracing how frames emerge can also reveal which actors in a policy field possess sufficient material and symbolic resources to impose their framing of an issue, and show how social institutions channel those resources. In other words, studying framing allows us to "tie [. . .] problem definitions to an analysis of power" (Vliegenthart and van Zoonen 2011: 108). A comparative analysis of the framing of health inequalities helps to denaturalize health inequalities, making it clear that they are not just facts "out there" to be measured and dealt with, but rather actively constructed as policy problems. We hope that this can encourage a deeper engagement with dimensions and causes of inequalities that might otherwise be missed, and may shed light on new ways to combat inequities.

We define health inequality policy frames as problem definitions, causal stories, policy prescriptions, and attributions of causal and treatment responsibility that can be detected in the form of key words, phrases, and analytic tropes in texts that contain the observations of the policy elites (researchers, policy advocates, bureaucrats, and elected officials) who constitute the health policy field.

We focus in this article on reports issued by national governments that deal either exclusively or in part with the problem of health inequalities, in order to identify the constitutive claims that national policy-making elites make about health equity: what qualifies as a health inequity, and why. Government reports are a standard source of information about how health policy elites understand health inequalities at a definitional level, and hence what policies are likely to be adopted in order to combat them (see, e.g., Docteur and Berenson, 2014; Graham 2004; Vallgårda 2007). Freeman (2006) articulates clearly the rationale for choosing to analyze these documents: "Government is a text-based medium, no less in public health than in other areas of public policy, and a feature of the politics of health equity across countries is that it turns on the production of a key text" (Freeman 2006: 52). The process of producing government reports on health inequalities helps to build constituencies for particular ideas and policies within the policy elite, as contributors negotiate over common language; the documents themselves become "a source of authority, a means by which influence is established and exerted, such that the production of the document may be thought of as a process of underwriting as much as writing" (Freeman 2006: 54; see also Raphael 2011).

Sampling: Country Cases. We selected three country cases for this comparative analysis. The United States, by virtue of the nature of this special issue, is the reference case. The UK in many respects constitutes a "most different system" comparison (Przeworski and Teune 1970). In 1998 the former British National Health Service was devolved into four autonomous units in England, Wales, Scotland, and Northern Ireland. Since then, there has been some divergence in the systems, particularly between Scotland on the one hand, and England and Wales on the other. The constituent countries of the UK nevertheless still all have single-payer, public national health systems that incorporate preventive and public health as well as medical care, and that provide medical care free or at low cost at the point of service to all legal residents of the UK and other European Union countries. As a result, policy makers in the UK may be more likely to consider the health system as an adequate tool for addressing health status inequalities, while at the same time inequalities in access to health care are unlikely to play as central a role in health inequalities discourse there as they do in the United States. Despite these differences, though, many policy areas relevant to health lie outside of the health system; and the UK is an important case for comparative analysis because of its outsized influence on the health inequality policy agenda throughout Europe.

We also consider the French case, which, in relation to the United States and in contrast to the UK, is closer to a "most similar system." Like the United States, France has a health system in which public health and prevention plays a very limited role compared to insurance coverage for medical care. Multiple public and private payers and providers constitute the medical care system, which, as in the United States, has led policy makers to be preoccupied with issues like the uneven supply of medical services, uninsurance, and cost-related barriers to accessing health care. Another important similarity between the United States and France for the purposes of this study is the political salience of race and ethnicity, which is clearly higher in the United States and France than in the UK (Crowley 1993; Maxwell 2012). Analyzing the framing of health inequalities in the United States and France together thus allows us to see how the politics of race intersects with health inequality policy frames.

Sampling: Reports. In order to assess the features of different health inequalities frames in policy discourses in the United States, the UK, and France, we conducted systematic qualitative content analysis, described below, of a sample of reports written or commissioned by the national government of a country that are mainly concerned with the issue of health inequalities during the period 1980 to 2012. This period begins with the release of the Black Report in the UK, which is widely recognized in the secondary literatures as the starting point for national-level policy attention to health inequalities in the industrialized democracies of the West. We end in 2012 in order to ensure that our search strategy, which depended in part on the secondary literature, would capture all of the relevant documents produced in that period.

To identify the universe of relevant documents, we first surveyed the secondary literature on public health and health policy in each country to construct a timeline including all mentioned government or government-sponsored publications; and we searched the websites of (a) the national health ministries, (b) any subsidiary organs that these ministries' websites linked to, and (c) the government publications offices to identify any additional policy documents related to health inequalities. Finally, we conducted Google searches for documents whose titles included the word "health" and variants on "inequality," "disparity," "difference," "divide," and "gap" in order to identify any documents that might have been omitted based on the literature and government website searches. From the lists of documents generated using these strategies, we then selected documents that met the following criteria: They are (1) "major" reports, that is, commissioned or released by the top level of the organization in question, rather than by a subsidiary department; AND (2) they are primarily concerned with health inequalities, that is, (a) the title contains the term *health inequalities* or *health disparities*, OR (b) the bulk of the report is dedicated to the problem of health inequalities. We also included major sections of general reports on the health system that were commissioned directly by the health minister, the national executive, or legislature and that met criterion 2(a) above. We eliminated any publications that met the above criteria but that were not "unified," that is, they were constituted by individual chapters on diverse topics relating to health inequalities and attributed to separate authors. Table 1 lists the sample of reports for each country.

Analysis. We identified the publication's date and producers (e.g., political appointees, national biomedical research centers) in order to contextualize the report and situate it within the broader stream of health policy

Table 1   Reports Included in the Analysis

United Kingdom	*Report of the Working Group on Inequalities in Health* (Black Report) (1980)
	Independent Inquiry into Inequalities in Health (Acheson Report) (1998)
	Dept. of Health *Reducing Health Inequalities: An Action Report* (1999)
	Dept. of Health *Saving Lives: Our Healthier Nation White Paper* (1999)
	Dept. of Health *Tackling Health Inequalities: Cross-Cutting Review* (2002)
	Dept. of Health *Tackling Health Inequalities: A Programme for Action* (2003)
	Dept. of Health *Health Inequalities: Progress and Next Steps* (2008)
	Dept. of Health *Tackling Health Inequalities: 10 Years On* (2009)
	Fair Society, Healthy Lives: The Marmot Review (2010)
United States	Dept. of Health and Human Services *Report of the Secretary's Task Force on Black and Minority Health* (1985)
	Dept. of Health and Human Services *Healthy People 2000* (1990)
	Dept. of Health and Human Services *Healthy People 2010* (2000)
	Institute of Medicine *Unequal Treatment: Confronting Racial and Ethnic Disparities in Health Care* (2003)
	Institute of Medicine *The Future of the Public's Health in the 21st Century* (2003)
	Dept. of Health and Human Services *Action Plan to Reduce Racial and Ethnic Disparities* (2011)
	Centers for Disease Control *Health Disparities & Inequalities Report (CHDIR)* (2011)
France	Ministry of Social Affairs *Les inégalités devant la santé: rapport de mission* [Inequalities in health: report of the commission] (1984)
	Haut Conseil de la Santé Publique *Allocation régionale des ressources et réduction des inégalités de santé* [Regional allocation of resources and reduction of health inequalities] (1998)
	Haut Conseil de la Santé Publique *Les inégalités sociales de santé: sortir de la fatalité* [Social inequalities in health: Escape from fatalism] (2009)
	Inspection générale des affaires sociales. *Les inégalités sociales de santé: déterminants sociaux et modèles d'action.* [Social inequalities in health: Social determinants and models of action] (2011)

and political events in each country. We then conducted a systematic close reading of each report according to a set of preestablished criteria (Appendix). Our reading focused on whether health inequalities referred, in each report, to differences in health status and/or differences in health care (*outcomes*); over which *groups* (e.g., by socioeconomic status, racial and ethnic categories, gender, disability status, geographic designations) the inequalities occurred; and whether different frames were associated with different language, for example, "difference," "inequity," and "disparity"—terms that convey different degrees of moral charge. We next turned to examining the underlying causal explanations and proposed policy remedies for health inequalities. Causal explanations for health inequalities tap into policy makers' understanding of the true drivers of health equity. Policy recommendations indicate the practical response of governments, but could be contingent on particular factors such as program renewals, the fiscal climate, or the proximity of targets. Summaries of the results of the analysis of the text and figures in these reports are presented in tables 2 and 3.

Results

United Kingdom. We begin our analysis of the framing of health inequalities with the landmark British document released in 1980, the Black Report. Commissioned by a Labour government, the Black Report was delivered to the incoming Conservative Thatcher government. Under the Conservatives there were no significant government or commissioned reports on health inequality, and the issue was only taken up again in 1998 when the incoming Labour government commissioned the Acheson Report. Over the course of the next ten years, Labour's health ministry followed up on the Acheson Report with a series of documents outlining a policy response and tracking progress toward the goal of reducing health inequalities. In 1999 the government released the *Saving Lives* public health white paper and outlined a policy program aimed specifically at health inequalities in *Reducing Health Inequalities: An Action Report*, and in 2002 the government established an inter-ministerial "Cross-Cutting Review" to summarize progress to date and outline a long-term policy agenda. The 2003 document *Tackling Health Inequalities: A Programme for Action*, which included a foreword from Prime Minister Tony Blair, laid out a plan to achieve the national targets for 2010 of reducing inequalities in infant mortality and raising life expectancy faster for the most disadvantaged part of the population. Five years later, in *Health*

Table 2 Summary Analysis of Frames Utilized in Analyzed Reports

United Kingdom

Report (pp.)	Year	Outcome	Language	Main groups	Causes	Recommendations
Black Report (329 pp.)	1980	Health	Inequalities	SES	Class inequality	Comprehensive anti-poverty strategy
Acheson Report (146 pp.)	1988	Health	Inequalities	SES	Socioeconomic positions	Reduce poverty, downstream SDOH
Saving Lives White Paper (165 pp.)	1999	Health	Inequalities	SES	Social conditions and individual choices	Reduce poverty and unemployment, work on downstream SDOH, change behaviors
Reducing HI Action Report (43 pp.)	1999	Health	Inequalities	SES	Not specified	Downstream SDOH, behaviors
Cross-Cutting Review (67 pp.)	2002	Health	Inequalities	SES	Social inequality	Reduce poverty, improve access to HC services, downstream SDOH, behaviors. Whole of government approach.
Tackling HI Action Programme (84 pp.)	2003	Health	Inequalities	SES	Social determinants	In theory and long-term, upstream SDOH; in practice and short-term, downstream SDOH and behaviors

Table 2 (*continued*)

United Kingdom

Report (pp.)	Year	Outcome	Language	Main groups	Causes	Recommendations
HI: Progress and Next Steps (88 pp.)	2008	Health	Inequalities	SES	Social inequality, SDOH, individual choices	Access to health care, early years, promote equality
Tackling HI: 10 Years On (147 pp.)	2009	Health	Inequalities	SES	SDOH, one mention of income inequality and markets as drivers of HI	Poverty, downstream SDOH, behaviors
Marmot Review (242 pp.)	2010	Health	Inequalities	SES	"Fundamental causes," "inequities in money, power and resources," SDOH as "causes of causes"	Poverty, downstream determinants, behaviors (but explicitly as residual solution)

United States

Report (pp.)	Year	Outcome	Language	Main groups	Causes	Recommendations
Heckler Report (239 pp.)	1985	Health	Disparities	Race	Disease-specific factors and social characteristics	Focused on health care; and research

(continued)

Table 2 Summary Analysis of Frames Utilized in Analyzed Reports (*continued*)

United States

Report (pp.)	Year	Outcome	Language	Main groups	Causes	Recommendations
Healthy People 2000 (692 pp.)	1990	Health	Disparities	SES, Race, Disability	Personal responsibility, poverty, medical care	Health promotion and prevention; multi-stakeholder partnerships; and data collection
Healthy People 2010 (62 pp.)	2000	Health	Disparities	Race, gender, disability, SES, geography	SDOH, access to care	Mostly disease-specific interventions and health care policies
Unequal Treatment (764 pp.)	2003	Health care	Disparities	Race, gender, SES	Discrimination, access to care, quality of care	Mostly provider-focused; and data collection
Future of the Public's Health (509 pp.)	2003	Health	Disparities (dominant)	Race, gender, SES	SDOH	Public health infrastructure; health care delivery; engagement from communities, employers, the media, and researchers

Table 2 (*continued*)

United States

Report (pp.)	Year	Outcome	Language	Main groups	Causes	Recommendations
HHS Action Plan (46 pp.)	2011	Health and Health Care	Disparities	Race	Social conditions	Mostly focused on health care; and data collection
CDC Supplement (113 pp.)	2011	Health	Disparities (dominant)	Race, SES	Social inequalities	Both health and social programs

France

Report (pp.)	Year	Outcome	Language	Main groups	Causes	Recommendations
LeRoux report (140 pp.)	1985	Health and health care	Inequalities, disparities	Geography, SES	Health care access, working conditions, unemployment	Improve geographic access to health care, reduce cost barriers, health care interventions, workplace health initiatives (incl. worker participation), intervention in rural areas *(continued)*

Table 2 Summary Analysis of Frames Utilized in Analyzed Reports *(continued)*

France

Report (pp.)	Year	Outcome	Language	Main groups	Causes	Recommendations
HCSP Allocation régionale (189 pp.)	1998	Health and health care	Inequalities, disparities	Geography	Health care access and quality	Improve allocation of health care resources according to need
HCSP Sortir de la fatalité (99 pp.)	2009	Health	Inequalities	SES	SDOH, health behaviors (structured by policy environment), cost barriers to HC access, contextual inequalities related to territorial policies	No specific policy recommendations beyond fact-finding, political will, cooperation across levels and branches of government
IGAS report (124 pp.)	2011	Health	Inequalities	SES, geography, gender	SDOH, health behaviors (as structured by policy environment)	No specific policy recommendations beyond fact-finding, political will, cooperation across levels and branches of government

Table 3 Number of Figures (Tables, Charts, Graphs, and Maps) in Which Health Inequalities by Selected Groups Are Depicted

	Report (pp.)	Year	SES	Race/ Ethnicity	Gender	Geography
UK	Black Report (329 pp.)	1980	17		6	2
	Acheson Report (146 pp.)	1988	5		6	4
	Saving Lives White Paper (165 pp.)	1999	6	2		2
	Reducing HI Action Report (43 pp.)	1999				
	Cross-Cutting Review (67 pp.)	2002	8	1	2	3
	Tackling HI Action Programme (84 pp.)	2003	1			
	HI: Progress and Next Steps (88 pp.)	2008	2	1		2
	Tackling HI: 10 Years On (147 pp.)	2009	11	2	6	
	Marmot Review (242 pp.)	2010	10		3	8
UK Totals			*60*	*6*	*23*	*21*
US	Heckler Report (239 pp.)	1985		24	14	
	Healthy People 2000 (692 pp.)	1990	6	22	6	
	Healthy People 2010 (62 pp.)	2000	1		1	
	Unequal Treatment (764 pp.)	2003		18		1
	Future of the Public's Health (509 pp.)	2003	1			2
	HHS Action Plan (46 pp.)	2011				
	CDC Supplement (113 pp.)	2011	15	18	13	13
US Totals			*23*	*82*	*34*	*16*
France	LeRoux report (140 pp.)	1985	21			7
	HCSP Allocation régionale (189 pp.)	1998				61
	HCSP Sortir de la fatalité (99 pp.)	2009	2			
	IGAS report (124 pp.)	2011	1			
France Totals			*24*	*0*	*0*	*68*

Inequalities: Progress and Next Steps, the Department of Health refined its policy response in light of slower-than-expected progress toward meeting the 2010 targets.

In 2009 the government commissioned Sir Michael Marmot to conduct an evaluation of the previous ten years of policy efforts, summarized in *Tackling Health Inequalities: 10 Years On*. With the exhausting of the national targets in 2010, the government commissioned another independent review on health inequalities, again tapping Sir Michael Marmot to lead the commission that resulted in the Marmot Review. This review, like the Black Report, was commissioned by a Labour government but delivered to a Conservative one. The incoming Conservative government published its own public health white paper in 2010, but it did not contain a sustained emphasis on health inequalities, and hence was not included in our sample.

All of the British reports focus mainly on group differences in health outcomes, mentioning health care only as one cause among many of inequalities in health status. The latter differences are uniformly termed "health inequalities" (not disparities, differences, or "variations," the term used by Thatcher's Conservative government after the release of the Black Report). While some of the reports reference health inequalities across geographic units (such as those between regions or health authorities within England), racial and ethnic groups, gender or disability status, by far the dominant group framing was class. For example, while the Marmot Review mentions "systematic differences" in health across gender and ethnic lines, the first sentence in the report, in the "Note from the Chair," states the main point: "People with higher socioeconomic position in society have a greater array of life chances and more opportunities to lead a flourishing life. They also have better health" (p. 3). Later in the Introduction, ethnic and gender inequalities are characterized as "additional sources of disadvantage and exclusion" that go above and beyond SES (p. 39). Furthermore, British documents rarely discuss the non SES-related drivers of variations in health status across regions or smaller geographic units. Small area variations, in particular, are consistently presented as a proxy for the effects of socioeconomic deprivation. Of all of the documents reviewed here, the 2002 "Cross-Cutting Review" alone stands out for having a sustained focus on geographic, ethnic, and gender health inequalities as well as inequalities defined by SES. Overall, attention to inequalities across racial and ethnic groups (6 figures), across geographic areas (17 figures, 4 maps), and between men and women (23 figures) each garnered only a fraction of the attention devoted to class-based inequalities (60 figures).

The cohesive focus on SES inequalities in British documents is associated with a similarly cohesive set of causal stories to explain the origins of these inequalities. The Black and Acheson reports both use a political economy framework to explain health inequalities, positing a through-line linking economic and social structure, the experiences of occupants of different classes (Black) or socioeconomic positions (Acheson), and health outcomes. Worse health among working-class people was not a result of unhealthy working conditions or insufficient resources alone, however; the subjective experience of low socioeconomic position had its own independent effects on health behaviors and health outcomes—a position reiterated in the "Cross-Cutting Review." Subsequent Labour government reports engaged in less pointed class analyses, but nevertheless assigned primary causal responsibility for health inequalities to underlying inequalities in "social conditions" or "social determinants." By 2010, however, unabated health inequalities justified a return to more politicized language. The authors of the 2010 Marmot Report drew freely on the language of the 2008 WHO report of the Commission on Social Determinants of Health (CSDH), which was also led by Marmot, to declare that health inequalities were a result of "inequities in power, money, and resources" (CSDH 2008: 16, 37), and even cited the Phelan, Link et al. (2004) theory of fundamental causation.

But, while some British health inequalities documents contained an implicit critique of market capitalism at the level of causal explanation, at the level of policy recommendations they were more muted. Despite references to the social gradient in health, some of the furthest "upstream" policy recommendations were aimed at reducing poverty and deprivation, particularly among children, rather than dampening income inequality more generally. Labour government documents after Acheson mentioned reducing income inequality as a solution to the problem of health inequalities, but in practice this meant only action on the very bottom of the income distribution (implementing a minimum wage, upgrading minimum income benefits for families with young children and the elderly, and adjusting taxes and benefits to incentivize work). These interventions did reduce the incidence of poverty, and together with investments in early childhood education and housing surely made a real difference for many families at risk of having poor health outcomes. But the policy recommendations were nevertheless at odds with the more trenchant underlying critique contained within the causal theories espoused by the authors of these documents.

United States. The first major report to be produced by the US government on health inequalities was *Report of the Secretary's Task Force on Black and Minority Health*, spearheaded by then-Secretary of Health and Human Services Margaret Heckler in 1985 (also known as the "Heckler Report"). The report is credited for first drawing attention to the issue of racial disparities in health (Docteur and Berenson 2014), which became a core theme of the agency's health strategy as outlined five years later in *Healthy People 2000* (HHS 1990). The strategy received a significant update in 2000 with the publication of *Healthy People 2010* (HHS 2000). Around this time, a key group of government consultants at the Institute of Medicine began devoting resources and attention to the study of health inequalities. Commissioned by congressional leaders in 2003, *Unequal Treatment: Confronting Racial and Ethnic Disparities in Health Care* was the IOM's first major statement on the issue of health disparities. The text self-consciously focused on differences in access to health *care* rather than health outcomes. It was followed in the same year by a report that placed greater emphasis on population health: *The Future of the Public's Health in the 21st Century* (2003). This report was a joint project of multiple health-oriented government agencies: the Centers for Disease Control and Prevention, the National Institutes of Health, the Health Resources and Services Administration, the Substance Abuse and Mental Health Services Administration, the Department of Health and Human Services (HHS) office for Planning and Evaluation, and the HHS Office of Disease Prevention and Health Promotion. The HHS *Action Plan to Reduce Racial and Ethnic Disparities* (2011) is the most recent update to the agency's policy strategy; and the CDC's January 14, 2011, supplement to its *Morbidity and Mortality Weekly Report* entitled *Health Disparities & Inequalities Report* justifies the Center's ongoing attention to the issue.

The American framing of health inequalities in policy documents differs sharply from the British one. American authors consistently write of "health disparities." *Unequal Treatment* and the 2011 HHS *Action Plan* include differences in health *care* as an outcome of interest, but label these differences, like inequalities in health status, as "disparities." *Unequal Treatment* defines the term as "racial or ethnic differences in the quality of health care that are not due to access-related factors or clinical needs, preferences, and appropriateness of intervention" (IOM 2003b: 20–21). Here, the link between disparities and racial and ethnic inequalities is patent. The link is less direct elsewhere, for example, in the CDC supplement, which defines health disparities as "differences in health outcomes and their determinants between segments of the population, as defined by social, demographic, environmental, and geographic attributes" (CDC 2011: 7). This more contemporary report also reviews the other language used to describe differences in health status, before ultimately settling on "disparity" as the operative language.

Despite the CDC's conceptual efforts to decouple the language of "disparities" from racial differences, the fact remains that health inequalities over racial and ethnic groups are the central frame in each of the US reports. Of the seven American policy documents we included, three reports are devoted wholly to inequalities across racial and ethnic groups (HHS 1985; HHS 2011; and IOM 2003b), and four reports make these inequalities a primary area of study (CDC 2011; HHS 1990; HHS 2000; and IOM 2003a). Compared to the British reports, the attention to race and ethnicity is staggering. However, it would be wrong to say that there is no attention to differences across other social groupings. Although the vast majority of tables, charts, and graphs in the American reports that illustrated a group-based inequality focused on race (82 figures total), attention is also paid to differences between genders (34 figures total), as well as across SES groups (23 figures total), and even across geographic areas (14 figures, 2 maps total). Nevertheless, major American government reports on health "disparities" always address race and ethnic inequalities, and directly or indirectly this term has acquired a racial charge.

Causal attributions for disparities in US documents are typically linked to social determinants. Whether the reports use this language and WHO's framework to explain these determinants varies. *Healthy People 2010*, the *Future of the Public's Health in the 21st Century* (2003), and the CDC supplement (CDC 2011) use the language of "determinants." Yet, both the oldest (HHS 1985 [also referred to as the "Heckler Report"]) and most recent (HHS 2011) reports speak of "societal factors" and "social conditions" instead (pp. 16 and 4, respectively). This suggests that the introduction of WHO discourse in the intervening period has made limited inroads in American reports on health inequalities.

Moreover, the reports frequently follow these discussions of "upstream" determinants with discussions of the "downstream" determinants: namely, access to medical care (e.g., CDC 2011; HHS 2000), and factors specific to individual biology and behavior (e.g., HHS 1985; HHS 1990). In the case of the 1985 Heckler Report, the "social characteristics" responsible for health inequalities are largely tied to the health sector: demographics, health education, health professionals, health care services, and financing (p. 13). Biological and behavioral attributions, for their part, often underscore salient US social cleavages, even in the most globally oriented documents. For instance, the *Future of the Public's Health* devotes an entire appendix to the various models of health determinants, including the Dahlgren-Whitehead model. Yet, the preface of this report points to the fact that "factors interact in complex ways with each other and with innate individual traits such as race, sex, and genetics" (p. 16). One document, the *Unequal Treatment* report, includes discrimination as an important source of racial disparities in health care: "Consistent with the charge, the study committee focused part of its analysis on the clinical encounter itself, and found evidence that stereotyping, biases, and uncertainty on the part of health care providers can all contribute to unequal treatment" (p. 18).

Given the relative weakness of the social determinants causal story and the strength of health care system-related explanations in US policy documents, it should be no surprise that policy recommendations are almost always focused on health care policies (e.g., access to primary care, improved cancer screenings). Even *Healthy People 2010*, which explicitly adheres to a comprehensive "determinants of health" approach (p. 18), develops twenty-eight focus areas for policy intervention that are largely dependent on changes within the health care system. The report, like several other US reports (HHS 1985; HHS 1990; IOM 2003a), also looks to community-based and local actors to spearhead these efforts. Only the recent reports have alluded to more comprehensive policy solutions. The foreword by CDC Director Thomas R. Frieden to the Center's supplement makes a clear plea to improve "health and social programs, and more broadly, access to economic, educational, employment, and housing opportunities" (CDC 2011: 2). The second section of the third goal of the HHS *Action Plan* calls for the adoption of a "health in all policies" approach and the piloting of a "health disparity impact assessment" for selected programs (HHS 2011: 28), but these statements are buried deep in the text of the report. The dominant emphasis in the American reports is on behavioral and health care-focused interventions. As Secretary Louis W. Sullivan stated unequivocally in the foreword to *Healthy People 2000*: "health promotion and disease prevention comprise perhaps our best opportunity to reduce the ever-increasing portion of our resources that we spend to treat preventable illness and functional impairment" (HHS 1990: vi).

France. The first report on health inequalities in France in the modern era was *Les inégalités devant la santé*, authored by Sylvie LeRoux at the request of the newly appointed Communist health minister Jacques Ralite and released in 1985. The issue of health inequalities surfaced again in preparations for the eleventh national Plan (a working group prepared a brief on health inequalities included in the health system planning document *Santé 2010* [Soubie 1993]), but the next major report did not emerge until 1998. The High Commission for Public Health (HCSP) issued *Allocation régionale des ressources et réduction des inégalités dé santé* in response to changes in the health care financing system that were prompted by *Santé 2010*. It is noteworthy as the first report from the country's main public health body that uses the term *health inequality* in the title. The next HCSP report on health inequalities, *Les inégalités sociales de santé: Sortir de la fatalité*, came more than a decade later (2009), and is explicitly addressed to "social" (i.e., SES) rather than territorial inequalities in health. The most recent major French report on health inequalities that we consider was prepared in 2011 by the Inspectorate General for Social Security (IGAS), and is once again nominally directed at social (SES) inequalities in health. The authors of the earlier documents frame inequalities in both health and in health care as problems. Geographic differences in health care resources and spending are presented as injustices in their own right, particularly (but not only) when resource allocation failed to keep up with the differing health care needs of residents. Later documents focus more on health outcomes, but cost-related barriers to accessing health care were still mentioned as prominent causes of health inequalities.

France has a long tradition of social epidemiology, which one might expect would make SES the dominant frame for discussing health inequalities among French policy elites, as it is in the United Kingdom. Furthermore, since 1965, data on mortality by both socio-professional category and place of residence, collected by the French national statistics agency (INSEE), have been available to researchers. However, discussion of health inequalities in France since the mid-1980s has had a strong territorial emphasis, with the SES-centered language so central in the UK appearing less frequently. While French reports on health inequalities discuss both differences in health status across SES groups and parts of the country as "inequalities," the territorial frame is far more prominent than in either the UK or the United States.

Consider some examples from the earlier French reports. The LeRoux report details the health consequences of hard, lightly regulated labor in France's countryside, factories, fisheries, and office buildings, but the report is nevertheless deeply territorialized in its structure, such that each chapter devotes some or all of its time to describing geographic inequalities. The 1998 HCSP report begins by noting that there are large differences in both health and health care supply between the regions, with the north of France generally disfavored on both counts. The report concludes that the best way to reduce inequalities in health status between regions would not be through health care spending, but by "*une politique régionale*" that devotes supplemental resources to disfavored regions (LeRoux 1984: 23).

Later reports continue this trend, while nonetheless attempting to integrate them into the emerging international consensus (illustrated, for example, in WHO's CSDH report) that framed health inequalities as primarily occurring over socioeconomic groups. The 2009 HCSP report on health inequalities characterizes territorial inequalities as linked to social inequalities in health, arguing that "the geographic environment constitutes one of the determinants of health." However, the territorial analysis recommended and carried out in part in the report is at a finer-grained level than much previous government analysis in France—at the level of the community or neighborhood rather than whole regions. And unlike earlier reports, this one casts territorial inequalities primarily as containers for SES inequalities (SES inequalities are "anchored" in "*les territoires*" [pp. 76, 92]). And IGAS's *Les inégalités sociales de santé: Déterminants sociaux et modéles d'action* similarly reflects current WHO language on health inequalities—but the report goes on to argue that "public policies need to take into account the relationships that link social inequalities in health with other forms of inequality, above all territorial inequalities" (p. 22).

As in the United States, the French reports for the most part limit their concrete policy recommendations to actions in the health care system. The exception is the early LeRoux report, whose political context—the report was requested by a Communist health minister—perhaps encouraged policy recommendations focused on workplace-related interventions, including worker participation in oversight of health conditions. The 1999 HCSP report and IGAS reports, both of which drew extensively on UK and WHO expertise, call for increasing the knowledge base around health inequalities, generating political will to tackle the problem, and cooperation across government departments and levels to resolve health inequalities. But these documents do not recommend specific policy interventions outside of the health care sector.

Limitations

Given the resources governments devote to preparing major reports, they are the most likely of any form of policy discourse to be fully informed by the scientific literature; but, as Freeman (2006) points out, they are also selective: the process of producing government reports on health inequalities helps to build constituencies for particular ideas and policies within the policy elite, as contributors negotiate over common language. This selectivity is a source of bias, but we see this bias as highly informative. Major government reports are unlikely to use problem definitions or highlight results that are supported by only a minority of those scholars or activists who work in the area of health equity and are deemed trustworthy by the government agency producing the report. Such reports are also unlikely to promote policies or understandings that are at odds with the perceived direction of political winds. These documents are, in other words, political. No single type of text offers a complete view on how all actors in a policy field conceptualize the object of their work. Analysis of scholarly research publications, news media coverage, or the texts of legislative debates, for example, could provide information about how health inequalities are framed in public debates. We chose to analyze major national government reports, rather than the scholarly literature, public sentiment, or internal government deliberations from which they often draw inspiration, because national government reports make authoritative statements of the policy direction that a government wishes to pursue.

Another potential source of bias in our data springs from the time frame we consider. While the Black Report is generally considered an unproblematic starting point for analyses of contemporary government efforts to reduce inequalities in health, the endpoint of 2012 could be more problematic. Already by 2012 there was some convergence across countries in the language used in government reports, as we have seen. Further convergence might well be visible if we extended the time frame to more recent reports. For example, the Affordable Care Act could push health equity discourse in the United States toward a greater consideration of health outcomes, now that some of the most pressing health care access issues have been addressed. The 2014 French government's *Stratégie National de Santé* is more consonant with the standard WHO-Europe framing of health equity—for example, recommending an interministerial body to coordinate action on health inequalities—and less focused on geographic differences in health care access than in years past. Nevertheless, the gap between language and action persists, and discourse about health equity under the Conservative government in the UK has moved decisively back in the direction of emphasizing personal health behaviors and local-level initiatives.

Discussion and Conclusion

Our comparative results reveal important differences between national health inequality discourses, as well as the historical development of these differences. A first important difference concerns the use of language signaling group *differences* versus language that contains a more explicit moral judgment about the unacceptability of these differences. British and French reports use "inequality" as the default term to describe group differences in health and health care that are preventable and unjust. The most commonly used term in the American reports, "disparity," is also linked to a sense of injustice, through its resonance with Title VI, which rendered disparate treatment of racial groups illegal. However, the language surrounding these core terms in reports from the three different countries differs markedly, with more frequent and more urgent appeals to a sense of (in)justice and equity in the British and French documents than in the American ones.

A second important difference between the reports from the three countries concerns the dominant group used to illustrate or frame the issue of health equity. Since the 1980s, policy documents in the United States have put much more emphasis on racial and ethnic differences in health status than on differences across any other group. Meanwhile, British reports in the past thirty years have included only a handful of charts, tables, or graphs reporting differences in health status across racial or ethnic groups, and French reports have shown none. One possible explanation for differences in attention to different group dimensions of health equity across countries is that government statistics are available only, or primarily, for certain types of groups. The fact that in the United States we have better data on mortality and morbidity by race than by SES, for example, likely reflects the fact that (socially constructed) race has always been a highly salient fact about American bodies, while class is often regarded as less important and/or impossible to measure (Krieger, Chen, and Ebel 1997). Meanwhile, while official British statistics have recorded occupation for at least a century, data on ethnicity is only available starting in 1991 (only country of origin for foreign-born Britons was available from the mid-twentieth century). It may come as no surprise, then, that while race and ethnicity are central axes of comparison in US health equity documents, British health inequalities documents privilege class differences in health status. In France, where there are no government statistics on race and ethnicity to draw upon, socioeconomic inequalities compete for attention with territorial inequalities in government reports.

Data availability certainly affects what types of analyses are likely to be conducted and hence reported—but governments can and do make changes to policies about what types of data to collect. And even when new types of data become available, government reports do not necessarily use these data. The National Institutes of Health (NIH) Revitalization Act of 1993 required that data be collected in order to allow analyses by race and gender (but not SES), which led to an explosion of research and evidence on racial disparities in the United States (Friedman and Lee 2013). However, while the British census introduced questions about ethnicity in 1991 (White 2012), some local authorities recognize that the "collection *and use* of this data remains inadequate" (Greater London Authority 2010, emphasis added). Indeed, government attention to ethnic health disparities in Britain appears to be limited to selected local authorities, particularly in areas with high immigrant populations, such as London (Greater London Authority 2010).

To explain the inattention of the national government to racial and ethnic differences in health in the UK, Nazroo (2003) points to the influence of Michael Marmot's conclusions in a 1984 study of immigrant morality rates: "Published shortly after the Black Report had firmly placed inequalities in health on the research agenda, this study used a combination of British census and death certificate data to explore the relationship between country of birth and mortality rates. A central finding was that there was no relationship between occupational class and mortality for immigrant groups, even though there was a clear relationship for those born in the United Kingdom. These findings led to the conclusion that differences in socioeconomic position could not explain the higher mortality rates found in some migrant groups in the United Kingdom." The study (Marmot, Adelstein, and Bulusu 1984: 277), which predated the expansion of available data on ethnicity in the United Kingdom, effectively removed racial and ethnic disparities from the research and policy agenda in the longer term. Curiously, one could imagine the same study producing the opposite conclusion in the United States, where policy makers emphasize how the differences in racial and ethnic health are *not* explained by class.

Just as data on ethnic differences are available, but largely unacknowledged, in the UK, other countries have enough empirical evidence to shift their dominant frames but choose not to do so. For example, in the absence of official government statistics on race and ethnicity in France, other forms of analysis could provide significant insight into racial and ethnic disparities. Some researchers have used census data on country of origin for non-native born French as a proxy for ethnicity (Berchet and Jusot 2012).

Analysis of small-area variations in health, which is prominent in more recent French reports, could also serve a similar purpose, given the spatial concentration of ethnic minorities in France. The territorial frame has deep roots in French politics where, historically, concerns over the state's capacity to rule and service all parts of the territory evenly has been closely linked to concerns about equal citizenship (Lynch 2016), so the explosion of small-area analyses in recent reports is not surprising. What is, perhaps, more surprising is that French government reports do not explicitly link small-area variations in health to the racial/ethnic makeup of these areas, instead leaving it to the audience to draw their own conclusions about whether racial and ethnic inequalities are problematic or, indeed, even exist.

Why, then, do the frames in US, British, and French policy documents about health inequalities differ? And what do these differences tell us about the nature of health politics in these three countries? In this article we can do little more than speculate. But different conceptualizations of what "counts" as a health inequality worth reporting on in the three countries are, we suspect, related to the particular historical salience of different cleavages in society. In all three societies, health inequalities are framed in terms of the broader inequalities that are already most familiar in politics. The survival of the landed nobility and aristocracy in Britain has made the British "a people uniquely obsessed by 'class'" (Lawrence 2000: 307) and, by extension, class differences. The legitimacy of class conflict as a mode of politics is inscribed in the British party system, where the main cleavage runs between the Labour and Conservative parties. In the United States, race is, of course, the most salient difference, codified into law and statute in a way that class has never been. Finally, the key register in which inequality is expressed in France is not class, but territory. Territorial unity was a central issue in the formation of the French state and French citizens (Braudel 1992; Weber 1976), the lack of access in France's "deserts" to the amenities and privileges of the Parisian way of life has been a theme animating French policy since WWII, and the determination to remove territorial disparities became a cornerstone of postwar French policy, codified in successive national economic plans (Baudouï 1999; Lynch 2016).

Because class in the UK, race in the United States, and territory in France are the most familiar and most institutionalized cleavages, they are, we suspect, the most readily accessible to researchers and policy makers, and the most likely to be incorporated into inequality documents. It does not, however, follow that these familiar cleavages are the most important in terms of the size or kind of inequalities they generate. For example, France and the United States both have significant SES-related health inequalities that receive less attention than do racial (in the United States) or territorial (in France) inequalities in health. And in both Britain and France, there is evidence of racial and ethnic inequalities in health (e.g., Berchet and Jusot 2012; Marmot, Adelstein, and Bulusu 1984) that receive little attention from official national reports.

The inequalities that policy documents *avoid* discussing too thoroughly may point us to areas of particular sensitivity. As painful as it may be to "discover" racial discrimination in health care in the United States, regionally inequitable distribution of health care resources in France, or class inequalities in health status in the UK, these inequalities are in some sense less threatening than would be class inequalities in the United States, territorial inequalities in the UK, or racial inequalities in France, precisely because they are more familiar and better institutionalized. Government reports may or may not offer meaningful solutions to the familiar inequalities, but recognizing that these familiar cleavages exist is not inherently threatening, and may in fact serve as valuable signals to particular support bases.

Whatever the source of differences in the group definition of health inequalities across countries, they coincide in these documents with a third important difference: the causal stories used to explain why health inequalities exist. In recent years, WHO has downplayed the role of health behaviors and health care in producing health inequalities, in favor of a causal story highlighting the role of social determinants and underlying inequities in power and resources. Policy documents in all three countries have adopted this "political economy" frame at least in part, but to different degrees. In the UK documents, the class structure of society—and even in some cases the market economy itself—plays an important causal role even upstream of the standard social determinants of health model. In the United States and France, on the other hand, the health care system remains a central actor in the reports' causal stories, reflecting incomplete health insurance coverage and significant geographic variations in access to care in both countries for much of the period under study. American documents additionally point to the role of personal responsibility (e.g., HHS 1990), and even discrimination (e.g., IOM 2003b), in producing some inequalities, while explanations in the British and French documents more frequently refer to larger-scale structures (e.g., income inequality) and processes (e.g., *l'aménagement du territoire*). American government reports have not, by and large, adopted the framing of health inequalities as socioeconomic inequalities in health status caused by an inequitable distribution of resources and power in society.

Not surprisingly, in light of these different understandings of the causes of health inequalities, documents in the three countries also differ in a fourth important way: in their policy recommendations. While reports in all three countries refer to whole-of-government, health in all policies, or cross-sectoral policy-making approaches, the extent to which the authors of the reports in different countries make recommendations outside of the health care system is striking. British policy documents contain multiple, concrete recommendations for interventions to reduce poverty, particularly among children, and in areas such as the tax and benefits system, transportation, housing, and the like. French and American documents instead make concrete policy recommendations mainly in the arena of health care, for example, increasing access to preventive care, expanding take-up of cancer screening programs and health education, and reducing cost-related barriers to accessing health care. Some elements—for example, health in all policies, health impact assessment—of the standard European suite of policy recommendations for reducing health inequalities have appeared in recent American work (e.g., HHS 2011). However, WHO plays a marginal role in American health policy, and there is no supranational equivalent to the WHO Regional Office for Europe or the European Union pressuring the United States to bring its policies into alignment with the reigning paradigm in health equity.

Despite these important differences between the health equity problem's framing in the UK, the United States, and France, there is the single remarkable similarity that unites these policy documents. That is, not one of these reports—not even those explicitly recognizing the role of income inequality in shaping health inequalities—made a policy recommendation that would entail significant redistribution of economic resources or power. While poverty reduction appeared as a major theme of British documents from the Black Report onward, reshaping the income distribution in a way that would significantly flatten the entire socioeconomic gradient decisively did not.

At one level this is not surprising: Why, after all, would a government report seek to undermine the political economic system on which it rests? Even WHO's CSDH report, while it argued in general terms for redistribution, was nevertheless largely "silent on the topic of whose resources, and how and through what instruments" (Navarro 2009: 440; see also Birn 2009; Escudero 2009). Redistributing income or wealth downward, let alone altering the systems of production and accumulation that give rise to income inequalities, is a politically difficult demand in the societies of Western Europe or North America where neoliberal ideas and practices are dominant (Lynch 2017). On the other hand, it is worth bearing in mind that the British reports discussed in this article were all products of a Labour administration that explicitly recognized the role of economic inequality in producing health inequalities, and was strongly and publicly committed to reducing these inequalities. More generally, one might question why a government would go to the trouble of convening experts, gathering evidence, and releasing a landmark report on health equity if its leaders did not sincerely desire to address the problem. Viewed in this light, the mismatch between the theorized causes of health inequity and the proposed solutions in these reports is indeed surprising.

What further factors could account for the lack of congruence between the causal frame and the policy recommendations in all three countries? Bergeron, Castel, and Saguy (2013) point out that much of the framing literature has tended to assume that policy outcomes will be consistent with dominant frames. Discursive institutionalists, on the other hand, have aimed to "show empirically how, when, where, and why ideas and discourse matter for institutional change, and when they do not" (Schmidt 2010: 21). To Bergeron, Castel, and Saguy (2013), this implies that, even once adopted as dominant, a frame may not result in the choice of policy instruments that is coherent with the dominant frame. One possibility, then, is that the political economy causal frame meets none of the preconditions suggested by Bergeron, Castel, and Saguy (2013) for a close match between frames and policies. First, the main articulators of the political economy frame, epidemiologists and public health scholars, are well-enough integrated into health policy making to be invited to contribute to the report; but their expertise is seen as marginal to the process of politics. Hence, their policy recommendations may be ignored or downplayed during the writing up of reports in an effort to make the recommendations more politically palatable. Second, even health policy-making structures are organized around an ecology dominated by medical, rather than public health, actors (see, e.g., Smith 2013 on the English case). This serves to limit the reach of public health experts' recommendations even within the broader health field. Finally, the political economy frame itself implies a need for major institutional and political restructuring—in this case, significant redistribution of power and resources. These three factors, taken together, could well explain the mismatch between the causal understandings underlying the health equity frame and the policies that are ultimately recommended and enacted in its name. So, perhaps the silence of British, French, and American health equity documents on the topic of redistribution should not surprise us. Nevertheless, some redistribution may well be necessary in order to significantly improve health equity.

In this article, we have sought to shed light, through comparative analysis, on features of American public policy discourse surrounding health equity that might otherwise go unnoticed. Our government's most emphatic statements surrounding health equity have cast the issue mainly (though never exclusively) as a problem of racial disparities, and, while they have recognized the role of social determinants in shaping health, have nevertheless tended to focus on solutions based in the health care system. If we are to make strides toward greater equity in health, and not only in health care, we must go beyond the policy remedies currently envisioned in government reports. Not only must we act on the proximate social determinants of health like housing, transportation, or food availability. We must also demand that our political leaders put on the agenda the more politically risky remedies at which even European governments have balked, remedies that will fundamentally redistribute the underlying inequalities in power and resources across racial, ethnic, gender, geographic, and socioeconomic groups.

■ ■ ■

Julia F. Lynch is an associate professor of political science and a senior fellow of the Leonard Davis Institute for Health Economics at the University of Pennsylvania. Her current research concerns the politics and public opinion surrounding health inequalities in Europe and the United States. She is the author of *Age in the Welfare State: The Origins of Social Spending on Pensioners, Workers and Children* (Cambridge University Press, 2006), and of articles appearing in political science, public health, and health policy journals.
Lynch.julia@gmail.com

Isabel M. Perera is a doctoral candidate in political science and a fellow of the Leonard Davis Institute for Health Economics at the University of Pennsylvania. She studies health and social policy in comparative perspective, with a particular focus on mental health.

Acknowledgments

The authors thank Alyssa Kennedy and Alexandra Babinchak for their tireless research assistance, participants in the 2016 RWJF Investigator Awards in Health Policy meeting for their extraordinarily helpful feedback, and the coordinators of this special issue for their incisive editorial advice. We are particularly indebted to Jeb Barnes for his comments. We would also like to thank the numerous academic colleagues and health policy professionals in England and France who made time to speak with us and help us understand the health equity issues facing their societies.

References

Bardach, Eugene 1996. *The Eight-Step Path of Policy Analysis.* Berkeley, CA: Berkeley Academic. www.health-inequalities.eu/resources/glossary/.

Baudouï, Rémy. 1999. "L'aménagement du territoire en France, antécédents et genèse, 1911–1963." In *L'Amenagement du territoire 1958–1974: Actes du colloque tenu à Dijon les 21 et 22 novembre 1996,* edited by F. Caron and M. Vaïse, 10–21. Dijon, France: Éditions L'Harmattan.

Berchet, Caroline and Florence Jusot, 2012. "État de santé: Une synthèse des travaux français, et recours aux soins des immigrés." In *Questions D' Économie de la santé.* Paris: IRDES. www.irdes.fr/Publications/2012/Qes172.pdf.

Bergeron, Henri, Patrick Castel, and Abigail Saguy, 2014. *When Frames (Don't) Matter: Querying the Relationship between Ideas and Policy.* LIEPP Working Paper (18).

Birn, Anne-Emanuell. 2009. "Making It Politic(al): Closing the Gap in a Generation: Health Equity through Action on the Social Determinants of Health." *Social Medicine* 4, no. 3: 166–82.

Black, Douglas, Jerry Morris, Cyril Smith, and Peter Townsend. 1992. "The Black Report." In *Inequalities in Health: The Black Report and the Health Divide,* edited by Margaret Whithead, Peter Townsend, and Nicholas Davidson, 1992. London: Penguin Books.

Braudel, Fernand. 1992. *L'Identité de la France.* Paris: Arthaud.

CDC (Centers for Disease Control). 2011. "CDC Health Disparities & Inequalities Report." *Morbidity and Mortality Weekly Report* 60. Atlanta, GA: Epidemiology and Analysis Program Office.

CDC (Centers for Disease Control.) Health 2015. *Health, United States, 2015, with Special Feature on Racial and Ethnic Health Disparities.* www.cdc.gov/nchs/data/hus/hus15.pdf.

Crowley, John. 1993. "Paradoxes in the Politicisation of Race: A Comparison of the UK and France." *Journal of Ethnic and Migration Studies* 19, no. 4: 627–43.

CSDH (Commission on the Social Determinants of Health). 2008. *Closing the Gap in a Generation: Health Equity through Action on the Social Determinants of Health: Final Report of the Commission on Social Determinants of Health.* Geneva: World Health Organization.

Docteur, Elizabeth, and Robert A. Berenson. 2014. *In Pursuit of Health Equity: Comparing U.S. and EU Approaches to Eliminating Health Disparities.* Washington, DC: Robert Wood Johnson Foundation and the Urban Institute.

Entman, Robert M. 1993. "Framing: Toward Clarification of a Fractured Paradigm." *Journal of Communication* 43, no. 4: 51–58.

Escudero, José Carlos. 2009. "What Is Said, What Is Silenced, What Is Obscured: The Report of the Commission on the Social Determinants of Health." *Social Medicine* 4, no. 3: 183–85.

Freeman, Richard 2006. "The Work the Document Does: Research, Policy, and Equity in Health." *Journal of Health Politics, Policy and Law* 31, no. 1: 51–70.

Friedman, Asia, and Catherine Lee. 2013. "Producing Knowledge about Racial Differences: Tracing Scientists' Use of 'Race' and 'Ethnicity' from Grants to Articles." *Journal of Law, Medicine, and Ethics* 41, no. 3: 720–32.

Gollust, Sarah E., and Julia Lynch. 2011. "Who Deserves Health Care? The Effects of Causal Attributions and Group Cues on Public Attitudes about Responsibility for Health Care Costs." *Journal of Health Politics, Policy and Law* 36, no. 6: 1061–95.

Graham, Hilary. 2004. "Social Determinants and Their Unequal Distribution: Clarifying Policy Understandings." *Milbank Quarterly* 82, no. 1: 101–24.

Greater London Authority. 2010. *The London Health Inequalities Strategy*. London: Greater London Authority.

HHS (Department of Health and Human Services) 1985. *Report of the Secretary's Task Force on Black and Minority Health* (referred to as the "Heckler Report"). Washington, DC: US Government Printing Office.

HHS (Department of Health and Human Services, Public Health Service). 1990. *Healthy People 2000*. Washington, DC: US Government Printing Office.

HHS (Department of Health and Human Services, Public Health Service). 2000. *Healthy People 2010*. Washington, DC: US Government Printing Office.

HHS (Department of Health and Human Services). 2011. *Action Plan to Reduce Racial and Ethnic Disparities*. Washington, DC: US Government Printing Office.

IGAS (Inspection générale des affaires sociales). 2011. *Les inégalités sociales de santé: déterminants sociaux et modèles d'action* [Social inequalities in health: Social determinants and models of action]. Paris: La Documentation française.

IOM (Institute of Medicine). 2003a. *The Future of the Public's Health in the 21st Century*. Washington, DC: National Academies.

IOM (Institute of Medicine). 2003b. *Unequal Treatment: Confronting Racial and Ethnic Disparities in Health Care*. Washington, DC: National Academies.

Kenterelidou, Clio. 2012. "Framing Public Health Issues: The Case of Smoking Ban in Greece, Public Health Policy Framing Equals Healthy Framing of Public Policy?" *Journal of Communication in Healthcare* 5, no. 2: 116–28.

Kickbusch, Ilona. 2003. "The Contribution of the World Health Organization to a New Public Health and Health Promotion." *American Journal of Public Health* 93, no. 3: 383–88.

Krieger, Nancy, Jarvis T. Chen, and Gregory Ebel. 1997. "Can We Monitor Socioeconomic Inequalities in Health? A Survey of US Health Departments' Data Collection and Reporting Practices." *Public Health Reports* 112, no. 6: 481.

Lawrence, J. 2000. "Review Article: The British Sense of Class." *Journal of Contemporary History* 35, no. 2: 307–18.

LeRoux, Sylvie. 1984. *Les inégalités devant la santé: rapport de mission* [Inequalities in health: report of the commission]. Paris: Documentation Française.

Lynch, Julia. 2017. "Reframing Inequality? The Health Inequalities Turn as a Dangerous Frame Shift." *Journal of Public Health* 1, no. 8. doi: 10.1093/pubmed/fdw140.

Lynch, Julia 2016. "Class, Territory, and Inequality: Explaining Differences in the Framing of Health Inequalities as a Policy Problem in Belgium and France." *French Politics* 14, no. 1: 55–82.

Lynch, Julia, and Sarah E. Gollust, 2010. "Playing Fair: Fairness Beliefs and Health Policy Preferences in the United States." *Journal of Health Politics, Policy and Law* 35, no. 6: 849–87.

Marmot, Michael G., Adelstein, Abraham. M., and Bulusu, L. 1984. "Lessons from the Study of Immigrant Mortality." *Lancet* 1, no. 8392: 1455–57.

Maxwell, Rahsaan, 2012. *Ethnic Minority Migrants in Britain and France: Integration Trade-Offs.* Cambridge, UK: Cambridge University Press.

Navarro, Vincente. 2009. "What We Mean by Social Determinants of Health." *International Journal of Health Services* 39, no. 3: 423–41.

Nazroo, James. 2003. "The Structuring of Ethnic Inequalities in Health: Economic Position, Racial Discrimination, and Racism." *American Journal of Public Health* 93, no. 2: 277–84.

Phelan, Jo C., Bruce G. Link, B, Ana Diez-Roux, Ichiro Kawachi, and Bruce Levin. 2004. "'Fundamental Causes' of Social Inequalities in Mortality: A Test of the Theory." *Journal of Health and Social Behavior* 45, no. 3: 265–85.

Przeworski, Adam, and Henry Teune. 1970. *The Logic of Comparative Social Inquiry.* Malabar, FL: Krieger.

Raphael, Dennis. 2011. "A Discourse Analysis of the Social Determinants of Health." *Critical Public Health* 21, no. 2: 221–36.

Reed, Adolph L., and Merlin Chowkwanyun. 2012. "Race, Class, Crisis: The Discourse of Racial Disparity and Its Analytical Discontents." *Socialist Register* 48: 149–75.

Saguy, Abigail C., and Kevin W. Riley. 2005. "Weighing Both Sides: Morality, Mortality, and Framing Contests over Obesity." *Journal of Health Politics, Policy and Law* 30, no. 5: 869–923.

Schmidt, Vivien A. 2010. "Taking Ideas and Discourse Seriously: Explaining Change Through Discursive Institutionalism as the Fourth 'New Institutionalism.'" *European Political Science Review* 2, no. 1: 1–25.

Simon, Patrick, and Vincent Tiberj. 2013. *Sécularisation ou regain religieux: La religiosité des immigrés et de leurs descendants.* Institut National d'Études Démographiques Working Paper (No. 196).

Smith, Katherine E. 2013. *Beyond Evidence-Based Policy in Public Health: The Interplay of Ideas.* Basingstoke, UK: Palgrave Macmillan.

Soubie, Raymond. 1993. *Santé 2010: Rapport du groupe: "Prospective du système de santé."* Paris: Commisariat générale du Plan.

Stone, Deborah A. 1989. "Causal Stories and the Formation of Policy Agendas." *Political Science Quarterly* 104, no. 2: 281–300.

Vallgårda, Signild 2007. "Health Inequalities: Political Problematizations in Denmark and Sweden." *Critical Public Health* 17, no. 1: 45–56.

Van Gorp, Baldwin. "The Constructionist Approach to Framing: Bringing Culture Back In." *Journal of Communication* 15, no 1: 60–78.

Verloo, Mieke. 2005. "Mainstreaming Gender Equality in Europe: A Critical Frame Analysis Approach." *Greek Review of Social Research* 117: 11–34.

Vliegenthart, Rens, and Liesbet van Zoonen. "Power to the Frame: Bringing Sociology Back to Frame Analysis." *European Journal of Communication* 26, no. 2: 101-15.

Weber, Eugen. 1976. *Peasants into Frenchmen: The Modernization of Rural France, 1970–1914*. Stanford, CA: Stanford University Press.

White, Emma. 2012. *Ethnicity and National Identity in England and Wales: 2011*. London Office for National Statistics.

Whitehead, Margaret. 1991. "The Concepts and Principles of Equity and Health." *Health Promotion International* 6, no. 3: 217–28.

Whitehead, Margaret. 1992. "The Concepts and Principles of Equity and Health." *International Journal of Health Services* 22, no. 3: 429–45.

Williams, David R. 1999. "Race, Socioeconomic Status, and Health: The Added Effects of Racism and Discrimination." *Annals of the New York Academy of Sciences* 896, no. 1: 173–88.

Appendix   Qualitative Coding Scheme for Government Health
Equity Reports

A close reading of the government reports was carried out by the authors to
identify the following themes. Particular attention was paid to the executive
summaries, prefaces, and introductions to the reports when assigning weight
to various frames. Additionally, each figure (table, chart, graph, or map) in the
report that depicted an empirical relationship drawing on data was coded
according to the outcome(s) and group frame(s) depicted.

Outcomes
- Access to health care
- Quality of health care
- Health status

Group Frames
- SES (including occupational status, education, income, wealth, employ-
  ment status)
- Race/ethnicity
- Geography (comparisons within the country of the report)
- Gender
- Disability
- Other (e.g., cross-national comparisons)

Language
- Equity, inequity, justice, injustice, fairness, unfair, fair
- Disparity
- Inequality
- Difference
- Gap

Causal Frames
- Individual
    - Health behaviors
    - Individual choices
    - Risk factors
- Health care system
    - Access to curative care
    - Access to preventive care

- Structural
  - Health behaviors, individual choices, risk factors *with* mention of structures shaping these choices
  - "Social Determinants of Health"
  - Other mention of social determinants
  - Deprivation (poverty, exclusion)
  - Discrimination, individual racism
  - Causes of causes
  - Environment
  - Upstream causes
  - Underlying causes, "causes of causes"
  - Structural, institutional racism
  - Political economy (class structure, capitalism, inequality)
  - Fundamental causes
- Other

Policy Recommendations

- Health care system solutions
  - Facilitating access
  - Upgrading quality, appropriateness
  - Greater emphasis on primary care and prevention
  - Changing provider behavior (e.g., end discrimination, more attention to determinants)
  - Expand use of screening
  - Changes to medical social services (e.g., home care for elderly, disabled)
  - Other health care
- Behavioral change solutions
  - Health education and outreach (in schools, workplaces, communities)
  - Smoking cessation programs
- Structural solutions
  - Act on structures affecting individual health choices
    - Restrict marketing of food, alcohol, tobacco
    - Tax food, alcohol, tobacco
    - Restrict sales of food, alcohol, tobacco
    - Encourage availability of health foods
    - More opportunities, facilities for exercise
    - Other

  – Act on social determinants
  - Education (not health education)
  - Income (raise minimum income benefits)
  - Limit unemployment spells through training, activation
  - Housing
  - Transport
  - Pollution (air, noise, toxic substances)
  - Dangerous working conditions
  - Community participation/empowerment
  - Other
  – Act on economy
  - Minimum wage
  - Limit unemployment spells by incentivizing hiring, reforming labor market
  - Redistribute income (not just by increasing minimum income benefits)
  - Limit capitalism
  - Limit free trade
  - Other
  – Act on politics
  - Redistribute power
  - Reduce structural or individual racism
  – Other (e.g., collect more data)

Words and Deeds: Presidential Discussion of Minority Health, Public Policies, and Minority Perceptions

Daniel Q. Gillion
University of Pennsylvania

Abstract   What are the different rhetorical approaches presidents used to address minority health inequality? More importantly, how have the efforts of presidents impacted minorities' perceptions of health? I offer a historical perspective that describes the three major periods of presidential engagement in discussions of minority health since the 1960s. I couple this historical overview with an empirical assessment that introduces a novel and extensive dataset of every presidential discussion of minority health spanning five decades (1960–2016). This study finds that, since the early 1990s, presidents have transported their discussion of minority health beyond the confines of Washington, DC, traveling to speak to local communities throughout the nation that have a dispropor- tionate number of blacks and Latinos. Moreover, a presidential discussion of minority health leads to greater salience on this issue and thus increases public health awareness. This work suggests that presidential messaging on minority health provides a frame- work for minority groups to understand and discuss the health disparities that may plague their communities.

Keywords   minority health disparities, presidential politics, racial and ethnic public attitudes

The federal government has made much progress in addressing dis- crimination and inequality in America since the 1960s, however, an area in which inequality has persisted over time lies within the area of health.

I sincerely appreciate the support and resources provided by the Robert Wood Johnson Foun- dation and the Ford Foundation that enabled me to conduct this research. Any opinions, findings, errors, conclusions, or recommendations expressed in this article are solely those of the author and do not necessarily reflect the views of the Robert Wood Johnson Foundation or the Ford Foundation.

Journal of Health Politics, Policy and Law, Vol. 42, No. 5, October 2017
DOI 10.1215/03616878-3940459   © 2017 by Duke University Press

From President Johnson's discussion of discrimination in hospitals to President Clinton's discussion of the AIDS epidemic in black communities to even President Obama's discussion of the Affordable Care Act, presidents in the modern presidency have attempted to address minority health. In their attempts to do so, they have all had to wrestle with the looming racial tensions that are invoked when politicians broach the topic of race. While these discussions are at times contentious, the president has a unique opportunity to increase health awareness and improve the public's understanding of minority health disparities through political discussions. Given the persistence of health disparities in the United States, I ask what are the different rhetorical approaches presidents have taken in addressing minority health? Moreover, have these discussions impacted citizens' perceptions of health?

In providing answers to these questions, I highlight the benefits that stem from presidential health discussions that are linked to an open and honest discourse about race. In particular, this article develops a discursive government hypothesis, which contends that the political rhetoric of presidents can move beyond the walls of government to shape the social-political agenda of black and Latino organizations as well as everyday conversations in the minority community. Political discourse initiated by the president raises the salience of health and provides pertinent information on program opportunities, new initiatives, and important statistics that are relevant for the minority community once the political dialogue is framed in racial terms. The information provided by the president is at times filtered through the minority media and later establishes credibility that resonates with individual citizens' perceptions of health. Taken collectively, politicians' rhetoric on race emerges as a vehicle to shape minorities' cultural attitudes on health.

The theoretical importance of this work lies in establishing value in race-conscious dialogue in government. As a consequence, this work conceptualizes politicians as being more than just policy makers. Politicians are also conveyors of important health information for minority communities when the discussion is framed in terms of race. Many prior works have viewed the role of discussing race as being important for political elections or public policy (e.g., Mendelberg and Oleske 2000; Wilson 1990). I argue, however, that discourse on race is important for policy implementation because it provides a medium to alter citizens' behavior on important issues in which government has begun to play a larger role, such as health. The argument advanced here, therefore, has important implications for theories of deracialization, as this article demonstrates that the dialogue on race has tangible benefits that move beyond policy creation.

In what follows, the article begins with a brief review of the existing scholarship on minority health and the use of deracialized rhetoric in government, proposes a modification that highlights the benefits a presidential dialogue on minority health can have for the minority community as far as increasing the importance of health, and continues with a historical assessment of the different rhetorical approaches presidents used to address minority health in the modern presidency. The subsequent empirical analysis supports the theoretical claims that presidents are able to alter public perceptions of health. The concluding section outlines the critical role that the political discourse of the president plays in improving health awareness in the minority community.

Presidential Discussions of Minority Health: The Fear and the Benefits of Discussing Racial Inequality

In the post–civil rights era, federal politicians' explicit discussions of race— in which they highlight the black experience, racial inequities, or race-specific governmental programs—have come under heavy scrutiny by scholars and political practitioners. Instead of a race-specific agenda, some scholars and practitioners have pushed for racial transcendence and written about the positive attributes associated with deracialization or a race-neutral discussion. These benefits have largely been advocated in agenda-setting and electoral strategies.

The advantage of decreasing the discussion of race at first took the shape of electoral benefits. Advising the Democratic Party in 1976, Charles Hamilton (1977) believed that presidential hopefuls would have a better chance of assuming office if they minimized their discussion of issues that were only relevant to the black community and broadened their rhetoric to discuss issues that affected blacks and whites equally, such as unemployment. The benefits of running the kind of deracialized campaign Hamilton advocated have been seen outside of presidential politics. In a 1989 off-year election, for example, a deracialized approach helped bring about what McCormick (1989) refers to as "Black Tuesday," when several black mayors were elected to office and Douglas Wilder became the first African American to win a gubernatorial race (McCormick and Jones 1993). Even in congressional elections in the early 1990s, black candidates who ran a deracialized campaign and expressed moderate views on race were more successful than black candidates who only advocated for black issues (Canon, Schousen, and Sellers 1996). As a consequence, more political candidates have either shied away from a political discourse that addresses race or deemphasized its importance in political campaigns (Gillespie 2012).

A deracialized approach, however, does not end with elections. Political figures who run deracialized campaigns later support race-neutral policies or fail to support bills that target minority interests (Orey and Ricks 2007). Scholars have supported continuing this strategy of deemphasizing race, indicating that a race-neutral approach would mean a greater alliance of politicians who are willing to support universal governmental programs that disproportionately benefit the more disadvantaged members of minority groups (Wilson 1990). In presidential politics, some argue that even President Obama embraced this race-neutral approach and has benefited from it by achieving electoral successes (Harris 2012).

Although much has been written about the benefits of deemphasizing discussions of race, little is known about the societal value of retaining a race-conscious dialogue in government. This is because the debate around politicians' discussion of race has largely been framed with two goals in mind: politicians getting elected to office, and the successful passage of policies that address disparities. There are good reasons for scholars to focus on these facets of the political process. Elections provide an opportunity to place in office those individuals who can best advocate for minority interests. And public policies provide structural opportunities to combat the institutional norms that have historically hindered minorities from achieving equality. While political rhetoric can certainly have an effect on these two goals, it is also possible that the political dialogue on race has a more far-reaching influence on society's cultural norms.

One area where political rhetoric may have a more extensive reach is within the issue of health. Political scientists rarely study the politics of health. However, sweeping reforms to the health care system with the Affordable Care Act have catapulted government into the center of the health care debate. It has also forced politicians to create a political dialogue that communicates important health information to the American public and thus shapes public health awareness. The health information conveyed by government is important because the growing racial health disparity gap is coupled with a burgeoning information gap that exists along racial lines (Lorence, Park, and Fox 2006). The information gap has been shown to partially explain certain health disparities that disproportionately impact racial and ethnic minority groups (Goswami and Melkote

1997; Viswanath et al. 2006). The lack of health information is reflected in low levels of health awareness in the minority community.

Scholars have long advocated that policy makers become involved in the process of increasing awareness on racial and ethnic disparities in health care and with health conditions more generally (Betancourt and King 2003). However, politicians may need to engage in a discourse on race alongside their discussions on health in order to promote health awareness. Indeed, some argue that the most telling evidence of the inadequacy of a race-neutral or color-blind approach to governance has been found in health and health care (Wise 2010). In considering the best practices to discuss racial and ethnic health inequality, some scholars suggest that the messaging of racial health inequality should focus on social determinants of health (Kim 2010). Others push for a broad message that invokes interconnections and shared responsibility among citizens (Wallack, Lawrence, Park, and Fox 2005). Regardless of the approach, there is a large consensus that government cannot ignore the issue of racial health disparities.

I argue that when political officials talk about race they initiate a component of what I refer to as discursive governance. In discursive governance, politicians' statements have influence beyond the policy-making process. The political discourse on race permeates throughout influential minority institutions within the black and Latino public sphere that seek to set the agenda for the minority community. The minority press, like other minority institutions, is keen to the political dialogue on race (Knobloch-Westerwick, Appiah, and Alter 2008). The race-related political discourse in government allows minority institutions to see the implications that follow from public policy, examine how public policies have considered and incorporated the minority experience, and ascertain possible opportunities to influence government. When federal politicians discuss race with regard to a secondary issue, such as health, they add salience to the secondary issue and thus increase the likelihood that the minority press covers this topic. For health issues this is particularly important because it allows politicians, who are typically not considered providers of health information, to increase health awareness at the macro level.

Presidential speeches may have a direct or indirect influence on individuals. Presidents have often been viewed as opinion leaders (see, e.g., Cohen 1995; Wood 2009). The mere words of presidents have been found to change economic conditions and even consumer behavior (Wood 2009). Presidents' discussions of racial issues can place minority concerns on the public's agenda as an important topic (Cohen 1995). Recent research has even shown that when presidents speak about social issues in a context that references racial and ethnic minority groups, minorities are more inclined to view this topic as being one of the most important issues facing America (Gillion 2013). Given that fluctuations in racial minorities' political behavior and attitudes are shaped by governments' attention to the minority community (Dawson 1994), presidential statements on citizens' well-being that are presented in the context of race provide a frame in which the issue of health becomes more salient for blacks and Latinos. These arguments lead me to propose the following hypothesis: presidents' race-conscious discussions of health will increase the importance of health for racial and ethnic minority citizens. Before I proceed to test this hypothesis, I offer a brief historical assessment of presidents addressing minority health.

Historical Snippets of Presidential Approaches to Addressing Health Inequality in the Minority Community

Presidents' discussions of minority health can be categorized into three different eras. In the 1960s, presidents addressed minority health alongside the fight for civil rights. The 1970s and 1980s witnessed a more conservative approach to addressing racial health inequality. By the 1990s and 2000s, however, presidents not only returned to a more aggressive discussion of addressing minority health disparities, but presidents in this era took their minority health messages to local communities.

Addressing Health alongside the Fight for Civil Rights (1960s)

The health inequality that existed in America along racial lines was undeniable in the middle of the twentieth century. As David Barton Smith (2005: 317) assessed, there were three major challenges the federal government faced in the 1960s: (1) the broader practice of Jim Crow that separated black and white patients, (2) the less noticeable, subtle forms of discrimination pursued by physicians through referrals and also seen through insurance status of patients, and (3) the ability to give all patients nondiscriminatory treatment once they had equal access to care. Presidents Kennedy and Johnson decided to address these concerns.

In the years leading up to the height of the civil rights movement in the 1960s, minority health was not a major issue for the executive office. Indeed, President Eisenhower, especially in his last term in office, spoke very little on racial health inequality. This is not to say that health issues, more broadly, were not discussed. The efficiency of Social Security and medical care for the elderly were heavily addressed and greatly debated in Congress during the Eisenhower administration. Yet, these conversations rarely involved a specific discussion of minority health. However, John F. Kennedy's presidential campaign would be a major turning point for how the federal government discussed health inequality.

The Democratic Party's attention to the issue of civil rights provided an opportunity for Democratic politicians to speak broadly about racial disparities in America, including issues such as housing, jobs, and education. The inequities in minority health and well-being were also among those issues that were addressed. President Kennedy looked to address health inequality by providing racial and ethnic minorities equal opportunity to the health profession. Speaking as a senator in East Los Angeles on the campaign trail in 1960, Kennedy expressed some of these sentiments:

> If the full rights of our Constitution, the full values of human dignity, are not available to every American, then they no longer have the same meaning for any American. They no longer have the same appeal to those in other lands of other races and religions, and they are a majority whose respect we seek. And they no longer guarantee us a nation that draws upon the full talents of every citizen. We do not want a Negro who could be a doctor, in a city short of doctors, working as a messenger. (Kennedy 1960)

As President Kennedy went after African Americans' votes, he also began to consider their health concerns. By the time Kennedy arrived in office, his campaign messages turned into presidential remarks and executive actions. In a message to Congress, Kennedy exclaimed that he was directing the Justice Department to challenge the "constitutionality of the 'separate but equal' provisions which permit hospitals constructed with federal funds to discriminate racially in the location of patients and the acceptance of doctors" (Kennedy 1963: 229).

Kennedy's health messages had a racial component but these discussions were often couched alongside strengthening Social Security and medical care. This provided a broader appeal to the American public. President Lyndon B. Johnson continued this approach of speaking about race alongside broader health issues.

In less than a year after gaining office, President Johnson signed the 1964 Civil Rights Act. Title VI of the 1964 Civil Rights Act prevented institutions that received federal funding from discriminating against racial and ethnic minorities that required health care or medical assistance. Johnson would follow this legislation up with a strong push for Medicare. Johnson believed the link between improving race relations and medical access with Medicare was more than related to one another, but rather the success of one issue depended upon the success of the other. He expressed as much during the Inauguration of the Medicare Program, "Medicare will succeed—if hospitals accept their responsibility under the law not to discriminate against any patient because of race" (Johnson 1966).

By the end of Johnson's time in office, he touted that Title VI of the Civil Rights Act, as applied to Medicare, had significantly decreased discrimination in medicine with 95 percent of hospitals achieving compliance. He often offered the example of how half the beds in all-white hospitals were empty because black patients were sent to segregated medical facilities that were overcrowded. However, after a year of implementing Medicare, the half-empty hospitals changed their policies to admit blacks and were operating at full capacity.[1]

Johnson's attempts to address minority health did not end with Medicare. He focused on infant mortality rates and argued that he wanted "to reduce infant mortality, concentrating particularly on those minority groups whose death rates is [sic] highest." He also addressed nutrition and healthy eating habits in the minority community by informing the American public he had petitioned Congress for 50 million dollars to programs "designed to provide adequate nutrition for disadvantaged children." Johnson was a leader on minority health issues and supported programs that provided many benefits to the minority community. Over the next several decades, however, presidential rhetoric on minority health would be less supportive and more infrequent.

A Conservative Approach to Racial Health Inequality (1970s and 1980s)

After nearly a decade of liberal Democratic presidents discussing minority health equality alongside civil rights issues, the 1970s and 1980s witnessed a more conservative presidential rhetoric from the majority of Republican presidents that governed over this period of time. The conservative approach was exemplified by the degree to which Republican presidents spoke about

---

1. Scholars have indicated that the Medicare certification program Johnson implemented was instrumental in exposing and eliminating much of the racism that existed in the medical field (Reynolds 1997).

minority health, and their use of rhetoric that looked to restrict governmental funds for programs that disproportionately benefited racial and ethnic minorities.

Nixon embodied the former type of conservatism on this issue, and spoke less about minority health issues than his Democratic peers. However, on the occasions that Nixon addressed minority health, he pursued those issues that were pertinent to the minority community at the time. One of Nixon's major focuses was on sickle cell anemia. Nixon often cited startling statistics about this condition in the black community. In a Special Message to Congress regarding Health Care in 1972, Nixon indicated "about one out of every 500 black infants falls victim to the painful, life-shortening disease called sickle cell anemia. This inherited disease trait is carried by about two million black Americans" (Nixon 1972: 392). He later went on that year to sign the Sickle Cell Anemia Control Act, the chief provisions of which improved screening, provided information and education on the disease, and established grants to fund research that explored the diagnosis, treatment, and control of sickle cell anemia.[2]

While the 1970s saw a decline in minority health discussions from the executive office, President Ronald Reagan did not shy away from speaking about federal policies that were related to minority health in the 1980s. This increased discussion, however, cemented the conservative approach of constriction. Reagan focused his efforts on restricting and reducing governmental spending on programs that had previously addressed racial health inequality. Two programs that garnered the majority of his scorn were the nutritional benefits of the food stamp program and Medicaid, which he believed had engaged in wasteful spending. He exclaimed as much in remarks at the National Legislative Conference of the Building and Construction Trades Department: "The cost of food stamps went up by 16,000 percent in the last 15 years. Medicaid and Medicare—again, essential programs—have increased by more than 500 percent in the last 10 years. We don't have a trillion-dollar debt because you aren't taxed enough. We have a trillion-dollar debt because government spends too much" (Reagan 1982).

As a consequence of what Reagan perceived as wasteful spending, 400,000 families were removed from welfare programs at the state and federal level. In addition, requirements to qualify for federal benefits became stiffer. For example, individuals had to have less than $1,000 in

---

2. Nixon also put forth his own Family Assistance Plan to Congress and would pitch it as a way to bring about calm from the social unrest in the black community (Quadagno 1990: 15).

financial assets to qualify for public benefits, a substantial decrease than the $2,000 limit just a year before (Marable 2015). Marable (2015) argues that these cuts hurt the black community in particular.

A thorough assessment of the conservative era, however, should not lead us to conclude that the executive office was only stagnant or even obstructive in improving minority health. On the contrary, President George H. W. Bush governed over an expansion of programs and institutions meant to address racial health disparities. Bush signed into law the Disadvantaged Minority Health Improvement Act of 1990. Later that year, led by the ambitious efforts of Louis Wade Sullivan, Secretary of the US Department of Health and Human Services, the Office of Minority Programs was established in the National Institutes of Health (NIH) Office of the Director. In 1992, the Minority Health Initiative was launched and provided federal funds to programs that addressed racial health disparities. Nevertheless, although there was an influx of institutions and programs established to alleviate racial health disparities toward the end of the conservative era, H. W. Bush took a conservative approach in addressing minority health by rarely discussing this issue with the American public.

Openly Discussing Minority Health and Universal Health Care Reform (1990s and 2010s)

The election of President William J. Clinton ushered in a new and aggressive approach for presidents to speak about minority health. Most Americans associate Clinton's efforts around health and health care with his failed proposal to establish universal health care reform in 1993. For many racial and ethnic minorities, however, the 1993 health policy is overshadowed by other health initiatives. Five years after the Health Security Act, in a radio address on February 21, 1998, Clinton put forth his Racial and Ethnic Health Disparities Initiative to combat some of the startling health inequalities that had become prevalent in the minority community. His initiative targeted those conditions that disproportionately affected African Americans, Latinos, and Asian Americans, such as infant mortality, diabetes, cancer, and heart disease. The policy was sweeping and bold. It set a national goal to eliminate racial and ethnic disparities by the year 2010. The policy initiative was also well funded. Clinton earmarked $400 million to spur prevention and outreach programs.

The president engaged in a powerful discourse on racial and ethnic health disparities during this time period. And his rhetoric on race served as the impetus for a larger discourse on this topic that rippled through other parts of government. Secretary of Health and Human Services Donna Shalala later established a task force to discuss innovative approaches to addressing racial health disparities through existing federal programs. Surgeon General David Satcher, an African American and a graduate of the historically black Morehouse College, also launched a campaign to educate the public about racial health inequities as well as to inform Americans about opportunities to address these disparities.

The president's efforts to address issues of health continued throughout the year. By the fall of 1998, Clinton had turned his attention to the AIDS epidemic that was still unraveling in the minority community. Congress was already making efforts to combat AIDS, but Clinton wanted to amplify these efforts with his own discourse. On October 28, 1998, Clinton addressed the nation on this issue:

> Today we're here to send out a word loud and clear: AIDS is a particularly severe and ongoing crisis in the African American and Hispanic communities and in other communities of color. African Americans represent only 13 percent of our population but account for almost half the new AIDS cases reported last year. Hispanics represent 10 percent of our population; they account for more than 20 percent of the new AIDS cases. And AIDS is becoming a critical concern in some Native American and Asian American communities, as well. . . . The AIDS crisis in our communities of color is a national one, and that is why we are greatly increasing our national response. Today I am proud to announce we are launching an unprecedented $156 million initiative to stem the AIDS crisis in minority communities. (Clinton 1988: 2167)

Clinton's larger dialogue on health that incorporated references to racial and ethnic minorities was unprecedented in the executive office. While previous presidents had offered statements on health, few made a continuous effort to discuss the increasing racial health disparities in America or to recognize the most troubling conditions ailing the minority community. Based on the total number of statements in the *Public Papers of the Presidents*, Clinton dwarfed the rhetoric of previous presidents by speaking three times as much on race and health than his predecessors.

Clinton's aggressive approach to discussing minority health would later be emulated by President Barack Obama. On March 23, 2010, Obama accomplished a historical feat by signing into law the Affordable Care Act, which put in place comprehensive health insurance reforms and looked to make health care more affordable, accessible, and of a higher quality. In the lead up to passing this law, President Obama rarely spoke about minority health. Actually, previous research showed that, in his first two years in office, Obama spoke less about race more generally than his democratic predecessors (Gillion 2013). However, in the years following the Affordable Care Act, Obama increased his discussion of minority health and attempted to broaden the public's understanding of how health disparities in black and Latino communities should concern all Americans.

> I said then that if a young child is stuck in an overcrowded and under-performing school, it doesn't matter if she is black or white or Latino, she is our child, and we have a responsibility to her. That if millions of Latinos end up in the emergency room because they don't have health care, it's not just a problem for one community, it's a problem for all of America. When millions of immigrants toil in the shadows of our society, that's not just a Latino problem, that is an American problem. We've got to solve it. That's why we passed health insurance reform. . . . (Obama 2010)

Obama's discussions of minority health also moved beyond the issues of health care. He spoke about his White House Initiatives to address health disparities for Asian Americans and Pacific Islanders by promoting increased access to and participation in Federal programs. He discussed the harms of viral hepatitis, which disproportionately impacts the minority community. And similar to Clinton, he spoke about the pervasion of HIV in the black community, indicating that HIV infection rates among black women are almost twenty times what they are for white women. By the end of Obama's second term in office, his attention to minority health had surpassed previous presidents and was only rivaled by the extraordinary attention of Clinton.

An Empirical Approach to Understanding a Presidential Discussion on Minority Health

While the historical perspective is helpful in providing greater context to the discussion of minority health, we may gain more by charting this discussion over time and empirically assessing its influence. In order to further explore the link between a race-conscious dialogue on health and the response from the minority community, I rely on several datasets that provide information on the rhetoric used by presidents, and attitudes gleaned from individual-level surveys.

Like many scholars who explore race in sociology and communication (e.g., Bobo 1997; Coe and Schmidt 2012), I consider a broad definition of race that examines discussion of racial and ethnic minorities. In the post–civil rights era, the concerns and interests of underrepresented racial minorities have become linked. More importantly, presidents have come to use references to race and ethnicity interchangeably in the public discourse (Coe and Schmidt 2012). Not only have politicians broadened the discussion of race, but the attitudes and behavior of citizens have been shaped through a racial prism or racial hierarchy that includes the ethnic groups of Asian Americans and Latinos (Kim 2003; Masuoka and Junn 2013). Masuoka and Junn argue that, for issues with "clear racial undertones such as immigration policy, position in the racial hierarchy is the key feature to explain differences in public opinion" (2013: 5). Thus, I conceptualize a race-conscious dialogue as one encompassing references to immigration, Latinos, and Asian Americans.

Measuring the President's Dialogue on Minority Health

To examine presidents' statements that highlight health and race, I employ a well-established process of content analysis to assess electronic copies of presidential speeches found in the *Public Papers of the Presidents* series published by the Office of the Federal Register, which is a part of the *American Presidency Data Project* (Peters and Woolley 2015). While previous studies have focused only on major speeches such as the State of the Union Address to understand the president's discussion of race (Coe and Schmidt 2012), I incorporate an extensive array of presidential remarks that include public speeches, addresses, signing statements, press conferences, and comments in presidential debates, as well as State of the Union addresses. This novel data collection effort should increase our understanding of the messages coming from the president.

To examine presidents' remarks, I use the same classification process to separately code health-related statements and those related to race. The initial stage of the classification process required a training set to classify statements.[3] Scholars suggest that classifying 500 documents is sufficient for training programs, and as little as 100 can suffice for producing accurate results (Hopkins and King 2010). For increased accuracy, two research assistants separately read and classified a random sample of 1,200 paragraphs drawn from the complete dataset of presidential remarks across four presidents (1990–2012), with 300 paragraphs being drawn from each president.[4] For issues of health, the training set was classified into two

---

3. The training set is a dataset of speeches that has been classified by human coders and is then used to train computers to recognize health-related or race-related remarks during the supervised learning process.

4. The different presidents that were covered included Presidents George H. W. Bush, William Clinton, George W. Bush, and Barack Obama.

groups: statements that mentioned a health-related issue and those that did not.[5] For issues of race, the training set was classified into paragraphs dealing with race and those that did not. Identifying issues of health were coded based on explicit presidential mentions of health conditions, health insurance, governmental health programs, and even discussions of physical fitness and best health practices.[6] Classifying race involved explicit statements that included references to blacks, Latinos, Asian Americans, or minorities as a collective group. It also included mentions of racial disparities, racial discrimination, minority government programs, and broader discussions of the state of race relations.[7]

Having established the training sets, I use an ensemble approach that incorporates multiple supervised learning algorithms to classify representative speeches, a technique that improves the accuracy of classification (Grimmer and Stewart 2013, Jurafsky and Martin 2008).[8] Three different learning algorithms (general linearized models, maximum entropy, and support vector machines), also referred to as classifiers, were programmed by the training set and later classified the entire dataset of presidential speeches.[9] To validate the classification process, a fivefold cross-validation procedure was used to compare the training set with the computer-programmed classifications.[10] The interaction of health and race is simply those paragraphs that were separately identified as dealing with health issues *and* race-related issues. I refer to the intersection of these two paragraphs as being minority health statements or race-conscious health statements.

An example of a minority health statement comes from President Obama during a 2009 address to the NAACP Centennial Convention: "We know that even as spiraling health care costs crush families of all races, African Americans are more likely to suffer from a host of diseases, but less likely to own health insurance than just about anybody else." President Obama

5. All texts were pre-processed by removing punctuations, numbers, white spaces, and stop words, which are common words that are used so frequently that they have little informational value. The preprocessing produces improved estimates during the classification process (Meyer, Hornik, and Feinerer 2008).

6. While word order is often unimportant for quantifying text (Jurafsky and Martin 2008), our experience revealed that retaining the word order of health-related terms such as "Medicaid Benefits," "High Blood Pressure," or "Working Out," improved the performance of the classifiers. Thus, we include bigrams (word pairs) and trigrams (word triples) to retain word order.

7. Given that only explicit statements were used, the intercoder reliability was high at 95 percent and 92 percent, respectively, for health and race. The author was the final arbitrator of the conflicting statements and classified these remarks for the training set.

8. Incorporating as few as four different algorithms for machine learning correctly corresponds to human classification 90 percent of the time (Collingwood and Wilkerson 2012).

9. The program *RTextTools* in the statistical program *R* was used to classify the sentences.

10. The fivefold cross-validation process yielded 85 percent mean accuracy for overall minority concerns.

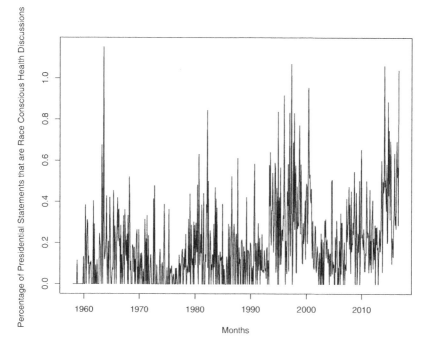

Figure 1   Presidents' Discussions of Health Issues in the Context of Race

discussed a broad issue, health insurance, which is not intrinsically related to race. However, the president intersects a dialogue on health with race by recognizing the racial disparities that exist for those who have health insurance. The coding process described above attempts to capture this interaction.

A more encompassing understanding of presidents' efforts to engage in a discussion of minority health is presented when we chart presidents' discourse over time. In fig. 1, I present presidents' discussions from 1960 to 2016. The unit of analysis is the percentage of minority health statements a president made in a given month. I consider one paragraph in the *Public Papers of the Presidents* to be a statement. Given this metric, the first point of note is that presidents rarely discuss health issues in the context of race, at least when we look at such remarks as a percentage of their overall discourse. At its highest level, such discussion made up only 1.2 percent of Clinton and Johnson's statements.

As one might expect, during the passage of civil rights legislation, Johnson spoke about minority health on several occasions and has the largest spike in a month out of any president. Other Democratic presidents displayed similar levels of discussion. While Republican presidents traditionally did not speak as much about minority health as their Democratic counterparts, Reagan was considered the exception. Reagan's discussions of cutting back on Medicaid and food stamp programs were just as aggressive as Johnson's remarks to eliminate discrimination in hospitals.

Arguably, the greatest level of discussion came under Clinton. In the two years before President Clinton came into office, George H. W. Bush's health statements were largely devoid of race-related issues. However, when Clinton arrived in office and made a major push for health care reform, his efforts for universal coverage included discussing racial health disparities. Though the proposal failed, it provided the groundwork for a larger dialogue on health and race that would come later in his administration. In June 1997, President Clinton announced his new race initiative that included the goal of addressing health care for racial minorities. Figure 1 shows its largest spike soon afterward.

After President Clinton, a clear pattern of deemphasizing race in health discussions emerged. President George W. Bush's discussions of Medicare and Medicaid, health issues he targeted during his time in office, often did not involve discussions of race. Although the dialogue on minority health improved with the election of the first black president in 2008, it was a moderate increase at first. Even with President Obama's extensive discourse on overhauling the health care system through the Affordable Care Act in 2009 and 2010, the discussion of race in his first term in office could not match the levels we witnessed under Clinton. Obama's second term in office is a different story. He aggressively discussed minority health issues and maintained this level of discussion for several years.

Not only can we assess the discussion of minority health over time, we can also explore the discussion across space. In fig. 2, I plot the places in which presidents engaged in a discussion of minority health. The figure is divided into two maps. The map on the top indicates the discussion of minority health before 1992, and the map on the bottom illustrates the discussion of minority health after 1992. It is clear that the discussion of minority health drastically increased across the country after 1992. Post-1992, presidents begin to transport their discussion of minority health beyond the confines of Washington, DC, to speak to local communities throughout the nation where there is a disproportionate number of blacks and Latinos. Cities such as Chicago, Philadelphia, Miami, and Houston have served as the epicenter for presidents to appeal to minorities about the importance of health. Although presidents are more frequently visiting these specific cities, the potential change in citizens' perceptions of health

Minority Health Discussion before 1992

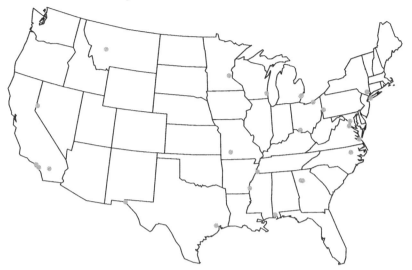

Minority Health Discussion after 1992

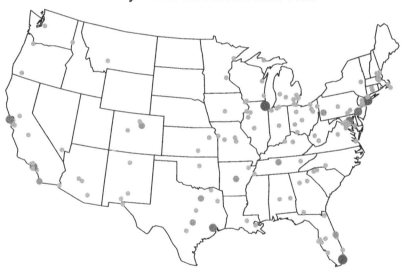

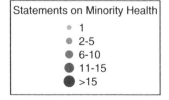

Figure 2   Geographical Location of Minority Health Discussion

in these areas could change the issues being discussed more broadly in black media outlets throughout the country.

As a consequence of this increased discussion in communities, we should expect there to be an influence of the president's words in a post-1990 era. We explore this proposition in the next section.

Individual Attitudes of Health Awareness

Thus far we have explored various aspects of presidential discussions of minority health. However, does the dialogue move to the micro level and change individual levels of health awareness? There are many ways to understand minority health awareness. We can conceive of it as educating the public on the benefits and consequences of health practices. Yet, the dominant narrative on minority health awareness is framed in a negative light, where the most discussed topics are, first, the lack of information society has on conditions that disproportionately affect marginalized groups, and, second, programs to remedy these disparities. Indeed, when presidents speak about health and race, they tend to highlight the racial and ethnic minority health disparities that plague American society or the inadequacy of health care insurance coverage among the least fortunate. These discussions are often a call for government action to mitigate these health disparities. Thus, presidents characterize issues related to minority health as potential problems facing America. As a consequence, when citizens receive these messages, they may also view health as a problem that must be rectified. If racial minorities recognize health as a problem, this may be interpreted as an indication of increased awareness.

In table 1, I analyze the impact that a presidential discussion of minority health has on citizens' perception of whether they feel that health care is the most important problem facing America. Various control variables are also included in the model to account for other possible explanations. On average, just 0.25 percent of presidential remarks in a given month relate to minority health. During those months that presidents offer an average level of minority health discussion, this only increases the probability that minority respondents view health as the most important topic by 1.2 percent. However, in months in which 0.65 percent of the presidents' statements were related to minority health, as was the case for Clinton and Obama, their discussion increases the probability that minorities view health as the most important topic by 7 percent.

While presidential discussions on minority health have a positive and statistically significant effect on minority respondents, non-minorities are unaffected by presidents' race-related rhetoric on health. In model 2 of

Table 1 Minority Health Discussions on Individual Responses of "Health Care" as the Most Important Problem Facing the Country

	Minority Response (Model 1)	White Response (Model 2)
President minority health discussion	1.140**	−1.78
	(−362.663)	(−195.929)
Age	−0.004	−0.007***
	(−0.003)	(−0.001)
Education	0.111**	0.013
	(−0.039)	(−0.013)
Female	0.471***	0.542**
	(−0.114)	(−0.035)
Obama in office	15.264	1.590**
	(−760.081)	(−0.579)
Presidential approval	0.171	0.347***
	(−0.168)	(−0.034)
Ebony articles on health	17.863	1.724
	(−760.084)	(−1.023)
Overlap of president and magazine	57.716	−8.131
	(−32.586)	(−14.692)
N	7554	72986
AIC	2868.431	27719.959
BIC	5363.171	31031.247
log L	−1074.216	−13499.98

Notes: Statistical significance is denoted as follows: significant at $*p < .05$; $**p < .01$; $***p < .001$.

table 1, the coefficient on presidents' minority health discussions is statistically insignificant. These results suggest that, indeed, certain political messages are interpreted differently by different segments of society. As previous research has shown, racial and ethnic minorities have a keen ear for a dialogue on race (Dawson 1994). Their attention to politicians' words is not diminished when the discussion of race is coupled with a dialogue on health.

Discussion and Conclusion

This article affords a deeper understanding of the benefits that stem from a race-conscious dialogue. Scholars often suggest there is value in discussing race but struggle to lay out the tangible benefits that follow from this discourse (McCormick and Jones 1993). This article demonstrates that presidents' race-conscious dialogue has positive cultural influences that move beyond elections and public policy to alter societal attitudes toward health and the agenda of minority institutions. The racial dialogue on health allows presidents to enter into the minority public sphere and shape citizens' perceptions of health, thus allowing presidents to become a part of deliberative democracy.

This article also offers a reconception of the role presidents play in addressing minority health awareness. For many, health awareness is information that is typically altered by primary care physicians, family members, or even the church. Rarely do politicians enter into this discussion. Nevertheless, with major health initiatives put forth by presidents since the 1990s, the role of government has come to be perceived as more closely linked with health. As a consequence, presidents are relied on to inform the public of important health initiatives that may combat the growing minority health disparities that exist in America. While research on how the political discourse relates to policy implementation and evaluation are often ignored, it is at these stages in the policy-making process that political rhetoric is most vital. Presidential communication can change citizens' reactions to governmental health programs. But even when new programs are not created, presidents can reshape citizens' attitudes toward health issues that exist in current programs.

Finally, this work highlights the importance of considering how race influences the entire political process. Even though a deracialized or race-neutral rhetorical approach may be beneficial for political campaigns and the passage of public policy, these approaches restrict an important pathway politicians may use to influence and engage with the minority community. For some issues, this engagement may be inconsequential. But for others, such as minority health and health awareness, it is an indispensable avenue of governance.

■ ■ ■

Daniel Q. Gillion is the Presidential Associate professor at the University of Pennsylvania. He was the Ford Foundation fellow and the Robert Wood Johnson Health Policy scholar at Harvard University as well as the CSDP Research Scholar at Princeton University. He is the author of *The Political Power of Protest*, which was the winner of the 2014 Best Book Award from the Race, Ethnicity, and Politics Section of the American Political Science Association. He also authored *Governing with Words: The Political Dialogue on Race, Public Policy, and Inequality in America*, which won the 2017 W. E. B. Du Bois Book Award from the National Conference of Black Political Scientists. dgillion@upenn.edu

References

Betancourt, Joseph R., and Roderick K. King. 2003. "Unequal Treatment: The Institute of Medicine Report and Its Public Health Implications." *Public Health Reports* 118: 287.

Bobo, Lawrence. 1997. "Race, Public Opinion, and the Social Sphere." *Public Opinion Quarterly* 61: 1–15.

Canon, David T., Matthew M. Schousen, and Patrick J. Sellers. 1996. "The Supply Side of Congressional Redistricting: Race and Strategic Politicians, 1972–1992." *Journal of Politics* 58: 846–62.

Clinton, William. 1998. "Remarks Announcing the HIV/AIDS Initiative in Minority Communities." *Weekly Compilation of Presidential Documents* 34: 2101–95.

Coe, Kevin, and Anthony Schmidt. 2012. "America in Black and White: Locating Race in the Modern Presidency, 1933–2011." *Journal of Communication* 62: 609–27.

Cohen, Jeffrey E. 1995. "Presidential Rhetoric and the Public Agenda." *American Journal of Political Science* 39: 87–107.

Collingwood, Loren, and John Wilkerson. 2012. "Tradeoffs in Accuracy and Efficiency in Supervised Learning Methods." *Journal of Information Technology and Politics* 9: 298–318.

Dawson, Michael C. 1994. *Behind the Mule: Race and Class in African-American Politics*. Princeton, NJ: Princeton University Press.

Gillespie, Andra. 2012. *The New Black Politician: Cory Booker, Newark, and Post-racial America*. New York: New York University Press.

Gillion, Daniel Q. 2013. *The Political Power of Protest: Minority Activism and Shifts in Public Policy*. New York: Cambridge University Press.

Goswami, Divakar, and Srinivas Melkote. 1997. "Knowledge Gap in AIDS Communication: An Indian Case Study." *International Communication Gazette* 59, no. 3: 205–21.

Grimmer, Justin, and Brandon M Stewart. 2013. "Text as Data: The Promise and Pitfalls of Automatic Content Analysis Methods for Political Texts." *Political Analysis* 21, no. 3: 267–97.

Hamilton, Charles V. 1977. "Deracialization: Examination of a Political Strategy." *First World* 1: 3–5.

Harris, Fredrick C. 2012. *The Price of the Ticket: Barack Obama and the Rise and Decline of Black Politics*. New York: Oxford University Press.

Hopkins, Daniel J., and Gary King. 2010. "A Method of Automated Nonparametric Content Analysis for Social Science." *American Journal of Political Science* 54: 229–47.

Johnson, Lyndon B. 1966. "Statement by the President on the Inauguration of the Medicare Program." Speech, Washington, DC, June 30, 1966. American Presidency Project. www.presidency.ucsb.edu/ws/?pid=27692.

Jurafsky, Daniel, and James H. Martin. 2008. *Speech and Language Processing*. Upper Saddle River, NJ: Prentice Hall.

Kennedy, John F. 1960. "Excerpts of Speech by Senator John F Kennedy, East Los Angeles College Stadium, Los Angeles, CA (Advance Release Text). " Speech, Los Angeles, CA, November 1, 1960. American Presidency Project. www.presidency .ucsb.edu/ws/?pid=25907.

Kennedy, John F. 1963. "Special Message to the Congress on Civil Rights. " *Public Papers of the Presidents of the United States: John F. Kennedy, 1963*. Washington, DC: Office of the Federal Register.

Kim, Annice. 2010. "Coverage and Framing of Racial and Ethnic Health Disparities in US Newspapers, 1996–2005." *American Journal of Public Health* 100: S224– S231.

Kim, Claire Jean. 2003. *Bitter Fruit: The Politics of Black-Korean Conflict in New York City*. New Haven, CT: Yale University Press.

Knobloch-Westerwick, Silvia, Osei Appiah, and Scott Alter. 2008. "News Selection Patterns as a Function of Race: The Discerning Minority and the Indiscriminating Majority." *Media Psychology* 11, no. 3: 400–17.

Lorence, Daniel P., Heeyoung Park, and Susannah Fox. 2006. "Racial Disparities in Health Information Access: Resilience of the Digital Divide." *Journal of Medical Systems* 30: 241–49.

Marable, Manning. 2015. *How Capitalism Underdeveloped Black America*. Chicago, IL: Haymarket Books.

Masuoka, Natalie, and Jane Junn. 2013. *The Politics of Belonging: Race, Public Opinion, and Immigration*. Chicago: University of Chicago Press.

McCormick, Joseph. 1989. "Black Tuesday and the Politics of Deracialization." Presented at the symposium *Blacks in the November '89 Elections: What is Changing?* of The Joint Center for Political Studies, Washington, DC, December 5.

McCormick, Joseph, and Charles Jones. 1993. "The Conceptualization of Deracialization: Thinking through the Dilemma." In *Dilemmas of Black Politics: Issues of Leadership and Strategy*, 66-74, edited by Georgia A. Persons. New York: Harper Collins.

Mendelberg, Tali, and John Oleske. 2000. "Race and Public Deliberation." *Political Communication* 17: 169–91.

Meyer, David, Kurt Hornik, and Ingo Feinerer. 2008. "Text Mining Infrastructure in R." *Journal of Statistical Software* 25: 1–54.

Nixon, Richard. 1972. "Special Message to the Congress on Health Care." *Public Papers of the Presidents of the United States: Richard M. Nixon, 1972*. Washington, DC: Office of the Federal Register.

Obama, Barack. 2010. "Remarks by the President at the Congressional Hispanic Caucus Institute's 33rd Annual Awards Gala." Speech, Washington, DC, September 15, 2010. Obama White House Archives. https://obamawhitehouse.archives.gov /the-press-office/2010/09/15/remarks-president-congressional-hispanic-caucus -institutes-33rd-annual-a.

Orey, Byron D'Andra, and Boris Ricks. 2007. "A Systematic Analysis of the Deracialization Concept." In *The Expanding Boundaries of Black Politics*, 325–35, edited by Georgia A. Persons. Piscataway, NJ: Transaction Publishers.

Peters, Gerhard, and John Woolley. 2015. "The American Presidency Project." www .presidency.ucsb.edu.

Quadagno, Jill. 1990. "Race, Class, and Gender in the U.S. Welfare State: Nixon's Failed Family Assistance Plan." *American Sociological Review* 55: 11–28.

Reagan, Ronald. 1982. "Remarks at the National Legislative Conference of the Building and Constructive Trades Department, AFL-CIO," Speech, Washington, DC, April 5, 1982. American Presidency Project. www.presidency.ucsb.edu/ws /?pid=42368.

Reynolds, P. Preston. 1997. "Hospitals and Civil Rights, 1945–1963: The Case of *Simkins v. Moses H. Cone Memorial Hospital.*" *Annals of Internal Medicine* 126, no. 11: 898–906.

Smith, David Barton. 2005. "Racial and Ethnic Health Disparities and the Unfinished Civil Rights Agenda." *Health Affairs* 24, no. 2: 317–24.

Viswanath, Kasisomayajula, Nancy Breen, Helen Meissner, Richard P. Moser, Bradford Hesse, Whitney Randolph Steele, and William Rakowski. 2006. "Cancer Knowledge and Disparities in the Information Age." *Journal of Health Communication* 11: 1–17.

Wallack, Lawrence, Regina Lawrence, Heeyoung Park, and Susannah Fox. 2005. "Talking about Public Health." *American Journal of Public Health* 95: 567–70.

Wilson, William Julius. 1990. "Race-Neutral Programs and the Democratic Coalition." *American Prospect* 1: 74–81.

Wise, Tim. 2010. *Colorblind: The Rise of Post-racial Politics and the Retreat from Racial Equity.* San Francisco: City Lights Publishers.

Wood, B. Dan. 2009. *The Myth of Presidential Representation.* New York: Cambridge University Press.

People, Places, Power: Medicaid Concentration and Local Political Participation

Jamila D. Michener
Cornell University

Abstract The geographic concentration of disadvantage is a key mechanism of inequity. In the United States, the spatial patterning of disadvantage renders it more than the sum of its individual parts and disproportionately harms economically and racially marginalized Americans. This article focuses specifically on the political effects of Medicaid beneficiaries being concentrated in particular locales. After offering a framework for conceptualizing the community-wide consequences of such policy concentration, I analyze aggregate multiyear data to examine the effect of Medicaid density on county-level voter turnout and local organizational strength. I find that, as the proportion of county residents enrolled in Medicaid increases, the prevalence of civic and political membership associations declines and aggregate rates of voting decrease. These results suggest that, if grassroots political action is to be part of a strategy to achieve health equity, policy makers and local organizations must make efforts to counteract the sometimes demobilizing "place-based" political effects of "people-based" policies such as Medicaid.

Keywords Medicaid, concentrated disadvantage, political participation

"Place matters" in profound, multitudinous ways and it is acutely consequential for those who inhabit the economic and racial margins of American society (Dreier, Mollenkopf, and Swanstrom 2004). The power of place is neither incidental nor innocuous. Instead, the social, economic, and political significance of where a person lives stems from public policies that create, contour, and reinforce systemic inequity. One way that policy does this is by facilitating the geographic concentration of people who are structurally vulnerable. Concentration is a mechanism through which

Journal of Health Politics, Policy and Law, Vol. 42, No. 5, October 2017
DOI 10.1215/03616878-3940468   © 2017 by Duke University Press

place-based detriments are distributed (Dreier, Mollenkopf, and Swan-strom 2004; Jargowsky 2015; Massey and Denton 1993; Rothstein 2014; Sharkey 2013; Wilson 1987). The density of disadvantage renders it more than the sum of its individual parts. A person who is poor and living in a community disproportionately populated by other people who are poor will suffer the deleterious consequences of poverty more severely than a similarly indigent person residing in an affluent area (Chetty, Hendren, and Katz 2016; Kneebone and Nadeau 2015). An analogous logic applies for race (Massey and Denton 1993; Sharkey 2013; Wilson 1987).

Evidence of this abounds in the domain of health. Racial and economic health disparities in the United States are powerfully linked to geographic context (Acevedo-Garcia and Lochner 2003; Auchincloss and Hadden 2002; Cattell 2001; Do et al. 2008; Grady 2006; LaVeist 1989; Marcus et al. 2016; Yen and Kaplan 1999). Counties, cities, neighborhoods, and states influence access to resources and demarcate exposure to risks. Public policies that concentrate disadvantage in particular ways are central features of the processes that link place to health (Ludwig et al. 2013). Advancing health equity will therefore require crafting, passing, and implementing policies that offset the penalties of concentrated disadvantage. Generating political demand for such policy should involve mobilization within the communities with the most at stake (Bambra, Fox, and Scott-Samuel 2005; LaVeist 1992; Schroeder 2007). However, concentrated disadvantage itself may influence the capacity for such communities to galvanize. Figure 1 illustrates the interrelated sociopolitical processes that connect policy, place, and political power.

Most of the pathways outlined in this conceptual model have been subject to empirical scrutiny (see relevant citations throughout this article). Social scientists of all stripes have authored voluminous explanations of the public policy roots of concentrated disadvantage (A). Sociologists have provided accounts of the relationship between concentrated disadvantage and health disparities (B). Political scientists have produced illuminating research about the democratic repercussions of public policy (E) and the effects of health for (individual-level) political participation (D). What remains underexplored is systematic study of how concentrated disadvantage structures political participation (C).[1] This article analyzes one facet of that topic by focusing on disadvantage channeled through *policy concentration*. After clarifying the importance of policy concentration and its relationship to both health equity and political behavior, I analyze aggregate multiyear data to

---

1. Two notable exceptions are Cohen and Dawson 1993, and Alex-Assensoh 1997; both are cited in this article.

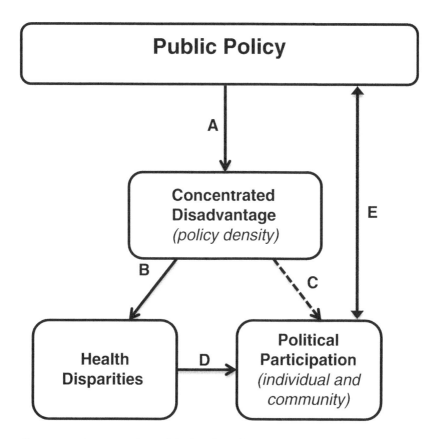

Figure 1 Conceptual Model of Policy, Place, and Political Power

determine how the concentration of Medicaid beneficiaries affects county-level political outcomes. I find that, as the proportion of county residents enrolled in Medicaid increases, civic and political membership associations decline, as do aggregate rates of voting. To the extent that political participation is imperative for achieving health equity, these findings suggest that we must pay close attention to the ways that "people-based" policies such as Medicaid (i.e., those targeted toward individuals with little regard for where they live) have "place-based" social and political effects.

Concentrated Disadvantage, Health Equity, and Community Participation

The concentration of disadvantage occurs when people who lack significant resources and/or bear substantial burdens cluster together in particular communities.[2] Such clustering enables "serial patterns of social contact and exposure that become crucial factors for how people construct interpretations of social reality" (Young 2003: 1073). This has ramifications for health equity. Health disparities are larger and more consequential in places marked by racial and economic segregation, even net of individual-level factors (Acevedo-Garcia and Lochner 2003; Cattell 2001; Do et al. 2008; Grady 2006; Marcus et al. 2016; Yen and Kaplan 1999). Though the full range of mechanisms that account for this has not been definitively established, there is little doubt that the geographic concentration of indigent people aggravates health disparities. From birth weight to diabetes to mortality, concentrated disadvantage drives divergences in health between whites and people of color as well as between affluent and poor Americans (Finch et al. 2010; Gaskin et al. 2014; Grady 2006; Marcus et al. 2016).

The prospects for progress on this front depend on cultivating the political capacity necessary to pursue policies that promote health equity. This is because "the biggest gains in population health will come from attention to the less well off," but policy change that benefits this group may be less likely to occur, "unless they have a political voice" (Schroeder 2007: 1226). Though it is certainly no panacea, political involvement from the bottom up holds promise for improving health equity. Even if the political engagement of those who bear the brunt of health inequities has only a limited direct influence on policy at the national or state levels, local political participation itself engenders collective efficacy, empowerment, and social capital, all of which are associated with improved health outcomes (Browning and Cagney 2002; Kawachi, Venkata Subramanian, and Kim 2008; LaVeist 1992; Ohmer 2007; Szreter and Woolcock 2004; Wallerstein 1992). Moreover, civically and politically organized communities attract health resources and disseminate health information more effectively than their less engaged counterparts (Viswanath, Randolph Steele, and Finnegan 2006). Overall, political participation is an important tool for improving health.

Still, participation is no easy fix. There are many reasons that low-income Americans are less likely to take political action: personal, institutional, and contextual barriers hinder their ability and motivation to participate, making

2. Sociologists have overwhelmingly focused on the concentration of poverty (Jargowsky 2015; Kneebone and Nadeau 2015; Wilson 1987). Yet, concentrated disadvantage is a broader concept because it attends to the clustering of aspects of economic vulnerability beyond poverty such as joblessness and "female-headed" households. Although such factors are correlated with poverty, they are distributed across geographies in different ways (Krivo et al. 1998; Massey and Shibuya 1995).

it less likely that they will "go to" politics (Alex-Assensoh 1997; Cohen and Dawson 1993; Hahn 2009; Pacheco and Fletcher 2015; Rosenstone and Hansen 1993; Schlozman, Verba and Brady 2012; Verba, Schlozman and Brady 1995). At the same time, the distance and disinvestment of mobilizing institutions makes it unlikely that politics will "come to" them (Michener 2016; Rosenstone and Hansen 1993). Public policy plays a notable role in these processes (and is also the result of them; fig. 1, path E) by shaping the dispositions and behavior of those who experience the benefits/burdens of government programs (Campbell 2012; Lerman and Weaver 2014; Mettler 2005; Michener, forthcoming; Soss 1999). One often-overlooked mechanism through which policy can operate is a phenomenon I call *policy concentration* (Campbell 2012: 340).

Policy concentration is a form of concentrated disadvantage that happens when particular geographic locales have disproportionate numbers of residents affected by a given policy. Of course, the distribution of policy across the population is not arbitrary. Even when policy is people-based, it is constrained and contoured by preexisting structural arrangements. Because of economic and racial segregation, low-income policy targets are often sequestered in particular counties, census tracts, or neighborhoods. Policy benefits/burdens are thus heavily concentrated in these communities. In an uncommon example of research that attends to this, Traci Burch (2013) shows that concentrated patterns of incarceration create communities from which residents (overwhelmingly African American and Latino) are disproportionately removed and imprisoned. Burch focuses on North Carolina and Georgia, where residents of disadvantaged neighborhoods experience imprisonment at ten times and fourteen times the national average, respectively (Burch 2013: 5). She finds that carceral concentration of this sort "diminishes the ability of all neighborhood residents to participate in politics," and she points to "social dynamics and economic resources" as the most likely mechanisms driving these effects (Burch 2013: 6, 9). In this article, I investigate the political upshot of Medicaid concentration and offer a framework of policy contact to explain why the local density of Medicaid beneficiaries affects the political life of entire communities.

Medicaid Policy Concentration

With more than 70 million enrollees, Medicaid is the largest public source of health coverage in the United States and the leading insurer for low-income Americans. It is the third most costly domestic program in the federal budget (following Social Security and Medicare), and the biggest source of federal revenue in state budgets (Paradise 2015; Rudowitz, Snyder, and Smith 2015). Recognizing Medicaid's immense significance, scholars have studied it closely, uncovering evidence that it has effects on outcomes ranging from mortality to mental health to educational achievement (Baicker 2013; Cohodes et al. 2016; Sommers, Baicker and Epstein 2012). Few studies have investigated whether and how the effects of Medicaid extend beyond individuals to communities. There is good reason to do so.

Geography is a key basis of heterogeneity in the distribution of Medicaid benefits. Due to the powerful institution of American federalism, states have been afforded immense discretion in fashioning the contours of Medicaid policy (Lukens 2014; Michener, forthcoming; Sparer 1996). By deciding the scope of eligibility, states exercise control over how large the program grows and what populations it covers (Andrews 2014; Sparer 1996). For example, in 2014, 54 percent of non-elderly Americans below 100 percent of the Federal Poverty Level (FPL) received health care coverage through Medicaid. But this proportion varied sizably across states: only 29 percent of North Dakotans below the FPL were covered, while 72 percent of West Virginians were.[3] Similarly, in Massachusetts Medicaid covered 68 percent of families without any full-time or part-time workers compared to only 30 percent in Virginia.[4] Parallel patterns hold along the lines of race and ethnicity: in Virginia, only 17 percent of blacks and 20 percent of Latinos were covered by Medicaid, while Iowa covered 53 and 41 percent, respectively.[5] These differences underscore the extent to which state decisions about policy design produce uneven concentrations of Medicaid beneficiaries across the country.

Comparable patterns exist for counties. Take California, for example, where county-level proportions of (adult) beneficiaries range from a low of 6 percent (Placer County) to a high of 31 percent (Modoc County). Some of this variation is straightforwardly explained by spatial differences in poverty and race, but much is not. For example, four very poor California counties include Kings, Fresno, Madera, and Tulare. These counties are situated in close proximity to one another. As shown in table 1, they have high poverty rates (between 21 and 26 percent), similar racial

3. Kaiser Family Foundation State Health Facts: Medicaid Coverage Rates for the Non-Elderly by Federal Poverty Level: http://kff.org/medicaid/state-indicator/rate-by-fpl-3/.
4. Kaiser Family Foundation State Health Facts: Medicaid Coverage Rates for the Non-Elderly by Family Work Status: http://kff.org/medicaid/state-indicator/rate-by-employment-status-3/.
5. Kaiser Family Foundation State Health Facts: Medicaid Coverage Rates for the Non-Elderly by Race and Ethnicity: http://kff.org/medicaid/state-indicator/rate-by-raceethnicity-3/.

Table 1 California County Comparisons

County	Medicaid	Poverty	Black	Hispanic	No English Proficiency
Kings	10	21	8.1	49.9	19.9
Tulare	20	26	2.1	58.3	22.9
Fresno	20	26	5.8	49.3	19.2
Madera	29	23	4.6	51.7	19.1

demographics, and comparable rates of English language non-proficiency. However, only 10 percent of adult residents in Kings County are enrolled in Medicaid, versus 20 percent in both Tulare and Fresno and 29 percent in Madera.

There are many reasons for these differences. California devolves responsibility for the administration of Medicaid to counties, so some of the differences in enrollment likely stem from heterogeneous approaches to poverty governance across counties (Sharp 2012; Soss, Fording, and Schram 2011). Since a confluence of policy choices, administrative decisions, and demographic configurations generate county-level variation in Medicaid density, these patterns are not a simple function of race and/or poverty. Evincing this fact: across all US counties, the bivariate correlation between the percent of adult Medicaid beneficiaries and the percent of African Americans is only 0.17, while the bivariate correlation with the percent of people living in poverty is 0.45. A basic regression model (not shown) predicting the percent of Medicaid beneficiaries in a county with controls for the percent of residents who are black, Latino, and below poverty (respectively), explains only 23 percent of the total variation. Insofar as the density of beneficiaries is (related to but) distinct from configurations of racially or economically marginalized populations, then Medicaid policy concentration may have a unique influence on local political behavior. Below, I submit that postulate to empirical scrutiny.

The Medicaid-to-Politics Link

The literature on "policy feedback" already provides reasons to believe that Medicaid is germane to political behavior. This body of work establishes that policies are not just an output of the political process but are also a critical input, structuring the relations among political institutions, government elites, and mass publics (Campbell 2012; Mettler and Soss 2004; Pierson 1993; Schneider and Ingram 1993; Skocpol 1992). Some of the most seminal work in this vein has shown that cash assistance programs, GI benefits, Social Security, and criminal justice policies influence civic and political participation by channeling resources, generating interests, and shaping interpretive schemas (Bruch, Marx Ferree, and Soss 2010; Campbell 2003; Lerman and Weaver 2014; Mettler 2005; Soss 2000).

Extending this literature, several recent studies have investigated how Medicaid affects political participation. Michener (forthcoming) shows that Medicaid beneficiaries are significantly less likely to register, vote, and take other kinds of political action. Importantly, this work demonstrates that the strength and direction of this individual-level relationship varies geographically: it is most pronounced in states that have recently reduced benefits and it is reversed in states that have recently expanded benefits. Complementing these findings, several other studies have identified an increased likelihood in voting at the district (Haselswerdt 2017) and county levels (Clinton and Sances 2017) in the wake of state Medicaid expansions spurred by the 2010 Patient Protection and Affordable Care Act.

Extending the work described above, I consider the theoretical relevance of Medicaid's concentration. I advance a simple but important hypothesis: *Medicaid policy concentration has community-wide political effects*. To clarify the logic underlying this claim, I offer a framework for understanding the channels through which Medicaid density might affect the political life of communities. I call this the policy contact framework (PCF) and describe it in detail below.

The Policy Contact Framework (PCF)

As shown by Joe Soss in his work on cash assistance programs, interpretive learning processes are a primary mechanism for policy feedback effects (Soss 1999, 2000). More precisely, public policies convey messages to beneficiaries that "teach" them about their political status and shape their political behavior. In this article, I emphasize that such messages are not limited to actual policy beneficiaries; they also educate those who encounter policy as a result of living alongside beneficiaries. Soss and Schram (2007: 122) make a related assertion, noting that, "participant status" does not define the scope of policy feedback effects. They astutely aver that, "participant status is only a particular form of a more general phenomenon: the experience of public policy as a visible and directly consequential factor in one's life" (Soss and Schram 2007: 122). I extend and build on this claim by focusing specifically on the role of place, and highlighting the mechanism of policy concentration as a means of making

Table 2   Types of Policy Contact

	Direct	Indirect
Personal	[A] Beneficiary (Michener, forthcoming; Lerman and Weaver 2014; Mettler 2005; Campbell 2003; Soss 2000) - Guardian of beneficiary (Levitsky 2014)	[B] Friend or family member of beneficiary (Walker 2014)
Impersonal	[C] Bureaucrat, school nurse, health aide (Watkins-Hayes 2009)	[D] Local community member unconnected to beneficiaries but hears about them via local networks

policy a "directly consequential" feature of community life. Policies can teach *entire* communities about government and politics. Quite crucially, however, the reach and content of such lessons hinges on how community members are positioned vis-à-vis two axes of contact with policy: (1) direct/indirect, and (2) personal/impersonal.[6] Table 2 summarizes the combinations of these forms of policy contact.

Direct and personal contact (box A, table 2) is what policy beneficiaries experience firsthand as they interact with government. This is the kind of contact implicitly theorized in most of the policy feedback literature. As far as Medicaid goes, such contact affects the political behavior of beneficiaries by teaching them contextually varied (but often negative) lessons about the capriciousness and (in)capacity of national and state government (Michener, forthcoming). Notice that the guardians of beneficiaries are also included in box A. This incorporates the parents of low-income or medically needy children and the adult caretakers of elderly or severely disabled persons. Although such folks are not typically a part of the policy feedback story, their experiences with government programs on behalf of the people they love can be transformative (Campbell 2014; Levitsky 2014). For example, sociologist Sandra Levitsky (2014) offers a compelling qualitative description of the distinct attitudinal feedback effects of Medicaid on middle-class caretakers who turn to the program to meet the prohibitively

6. After conceiving of this framework, I came across a distinct but related framework by Soss and Schram (2007). Soss and Schram focus on the dimensions of visibility and proximity, which do not overlap with the dimensions that I present here, though there are logical links between the two. The key difference is that I developed the policy contact framework described in this article with an eye toward understanding how policy affects *geographically defined communities*, while Soss and Schram focus much more broadly on how policy affects *mass publics*.

expensive long-term care needs of their elderly dependents. These care-takers tend to judge Medicaid by the expectations set via their experiences with (non-means tested) social insurance policies such as Social Security. In such a light, they usually find the program wanting and develop sharp criticisms, not only of Medicaid but also of related political phenomena (such as immigration and anti-poverty policies). The pertinent insight from Levitsky's work is that for Medicaid, policy feedback extends to non-beneficiary guardians who have direct personal contact with policy. Since such guardians are often part of the same communities as the beneficiaries they assist, they also increase in density as Medicaid beneficiaries become more locally concentrated.

Further expanding the scope of contact, the policy contact framework (PCF) next considers those who have *indirect personal* contact with Medicaid (box B). This includes friends and family of policy beneficiaries who do not have involvement as guardians (and thus do not directly interface with policies on behalf of beneficiaries), but who nonetheless have opportunities to hear about and observe the benefits and burdens that Medicaid brings. The political relevance of indirect personal contact is underscored by the recent work of Hannah Walker (2014: 811) who finds that "proximal contact" with the carceral state via someone connected to the criminal "justice" system has spillover political effects on broader groups of individuals who exist on that system's periphery. In the carceral realm, this includes folks like the aunt of someone who is incarcerated, the mother of a crime victim or the friend of a person who is unlawfully stopped and searched (Miller 2008). In the domain of Medicaid, analogous examples might include the parents of adult children who rely on Medicaid or the (ineligible) spouse of an actual beneficiary. Such people experience personal (i.e., connected to a loved one) but indirect contact with Medicaid that may shape their views of policy and politics. For example, in the 2015 Kaiser Family Foundation Survey, 27 percent of respondents report having been covered by Medicaid at some point in their lives, and 37 percent report having friends or family who have been covered (Norton, DiJulio, and Brodie 2015). Especially critical is that those with secondhand knowl-edge of Medicaid have distinct policy attitudes relative to those with no personal connection to the program. As shown in fig. 2, among survey respondents who noted having some connection to Medicaid (via family or friends), 70 percent agreed that the program was very important and 42 percent thought that spending should be increased (compared to 51 percent and 28 percent, respectively, for those with no personal con-nection). Crucially, vicarious connections are more likely in places with

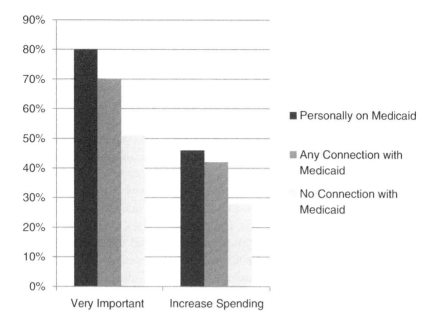

Figure 2   Medicaid Policy Attitudes by Personal Connection

high Medicaid density and are thus one channel through which Medicaid concentration might come to influence local political life.

Next, the PCF further parses types of contact by pointing to a group of people with *impersonal direct* ties to Medicaid: those whose employment brings them face to face with policy beneficiaries (box C). This includes (but is not limited to) bureaucrats working in local Medicaid offices, nurses staffing community health clinics, and home health aides taking on grueling and underpaid labor to provide medically needy beneficiaries with vital services. Though these "working class" constituents are generally beyond the purview of policy feedback studies, they are squarely within the reach of policy itself. As Celeste Watkins-Hayes (2009) shows, the people who do the work of implementing public policy are pushed to engage the political and social contexts that generate those policies. Moreover, in the course of fulfilling their duties, welfare bureaucrats exchange political ideas and draw on political beliefs that are reflective of their own race, class, and place-based identities (Watkins-Hayes 2009). The density of beneficiaries dictates the extent and nature of direct impersonal ties. As a result, Medicaid concentration may shape the political perceptions of the working classes that undergird the diffuse administrative apparatus of the program.

The final form of policy contact that I highlight is *indirect and impersonal* (box D). This includes local community members who have heard about Medicaid but have not dealt with the program or its beneficiaries in either a direct or personal way. Though they may seem too far removed to comment upon, people who fall into this category have numerous opportunities for meaningful policy contact, especially in a context of concentration. They may be connected to those who do have direct or personal contact (e.g., my brother's friend has a child that is on Medicaid). They may also be exposed to local messages targeted to beneficiaries (e.g., signs outside of health clinics urging eligible persons to sign up for benefits). More generally, since Medicaid finances many local services, the various institutions that rely on such funding may actively seek to shape the ideas of community members. Children's hospitals, medical providers, and other local organizations are potentially crucial intermediaries. For example, Texas Children's Hospital hosts a blog created specifically for the 12,000 "team members" it employs. This blog features regular pieces about health policy issues. On July 30, 2015, Mark Wallace, the president and CEO of the hospital, penned a post entitled, "Medicaid: Safety Net and Stepping Stone."[7] Wallace began by emphasizing how many people relied on Medicaid in the state of Texas and he attempted to convince his employees of the value of Medicaid to children and families. He said things like, "For me, regardless of my own political beliefs . . . I think about all the children and families who need our help," and "The simple truth is our federal and state governments save money by investing in health care for our children." At the end of the post, Wallace encouraged readers to contact their local political officials. As an elite positioned on the supply side of the health economy, Wallace used his platform to reach thousands of employees. Many of these people may not have had direct contact with Medicaid beneficiaries (either personal or impersonal), but they are likely to live in communities within driving distance of the hospital, and this is one example of how indirect and impersonal contact can teach key lessons about Medicaid.

A distinct but comparable process may occur when community members become the targets of local political officials. Budgetary politics in Rockland County, New York, illustrate this possibility especially well. In 2012, members of the Rockland County legislature voted for a bill that mandated a transparency measure requiring the inclusion of a separate line item for the "Medicaid tax" portion of local tax bills (previously, there was

---

7. See: www.onthemark.org/blog/medicaid-safety-net-and-stepping-stone.

a single item called "county tax"). This was intended to raise public awareness (and ostensibly ire) of the significant financial costs of Medicaid. Each year since the enactment of this legislation, tens of thousands of Rockland residents have received tax bills highlighting the "burden" that Medicaid places on them. Politicians leverage such communications to gain support from constituents. For example, a (now former) Rockland County legislative representative, Barry Kantrowitz, emphasized the encumbrance of Medicaid in a salient post on his website. As shown in the screen shot included in fig. 3, after noting that recent tax bills "included a breakout of the Medicaid expense as a line item," Kantrowitz devoted a section of his site to "tackling Medicaid fraud," pointing to his "efforts to prevent the abuse of Medicaid and other public assistance," and initiating provocative language about punishing "criminals." In this way, Kantrowitz sent a stigmatizing message to his constituents linking Medicaid to criminality. In view of such moves, opponents of the dual line policy now (quite reasonably) argue that it creates "resentment among our heavily burdened taxpayers about Medicaid."[8]

Though it is difficult to know how idiosyncratic the politics of Medicaid in Rockland County really are, they do not appear to be singular. A simple Google search turns up an example of another county in New York (Monroe) that devotes a separate line for Medicaid on local tax bills (see fig. 4). Moreover, since counties all across the United States have to contend with Medicaid costs to varying degrees, local officials have an incentive to mobilize constituents in opposition to the program, particularly in the context of policy concentration.

In sum, the policy contact framework helps to explain how Medicaid concentration can affect community political participation. For three of the four types of policy contact (direct personal, indirect personal, and direct impersonal), I draw on existing social science research to build the prima facie case for the expectation that contact will bear on political behavior (references included in table 2). The fourth type of contact (indirect impersonal) is not explored in scholarly research, but it is credible given examples such as that of Texas Children's Hospital and Rockland County, New York.

By delineating this policy contact typology, I provide conceptual support for the general hypothesis that Medicaid policy concentration has community-wide political effects. Recall that the mechanism I propose to explain this effect is an interpretive learning process by which experiences

8. See "Sticker Shock with 2016 Rockland County Tax Bill Wallop." Available online at: www.lohud.com/story/money/personal-finance/taxes/david-mckay-wilson/2016/01/21/sticker -shock-2016-rockland-tax-bill-wallop/79073846/.

BARRY S. Kantrowitz

Medicaid and your Property Tax Bill

Medicaid is a federally mandated program that requires states to provide medical benefits to those who qualify based upon financial criteria.   The term "unfunded mandates" refers to a variety of services and programs that are created by either the federal or state government but funded, partially or wholly, by the county governments. Only two states in the country pass the cost of the federal Medicaid mandate onto local governments-- Michigan and New York.

I was shocked to learn that in 2011, Rockland County's mandated share of the Medicaid costs completely exceeded the entire amount of the property taxes that Rockland County collected. That's right, 100% of all the property taxes collected in 2011 were not enough to pay the County's share of the Medicaid Mandate. In 2012, Medicaid consumed 91% of the property taxes received and in 2013 it was 80%. Medicaid costs have not gone down--- they have gone up-- but the County property taxes have gone up more. The 2014 budget projects Medicaid costs of $74,300,000 and property tax revenue of $105,060,167, which means that in 2014, Medicaid will still eat up more than 70% of our property taxes.

The 2014 State County and Town tax bills that were issued in late December and were due at the end of January included a breakout of the Medicaid expense as a line item. The expense was not new, but it was the first time it was shown that way on the bills. The purpose was to raise awareness of the cost of this mandated program.

Tackling Medicaid Fraud

As your representative in County government I will do what I can to speak out against the State mandates that are crippling our budget. I recognize however, that at least for the short term, they are here to stay. Therefore, I am supporting efforts to prevent the abuse of Medicaid and other public assistance by those who are taking advantage of a system that is overwhelmed. There are several bills presently pending in the New York State Assembly and Senate. I am sponsoring local legislation to encourage our State lawmakers to provide greater incentives to the county governments to criminally prosecute those that knowingly and intentionally defraud Medicaid.   By increasing the local government's financial stake in recoveries from criminal prosecutions, the number of prosecutions should increase. Medicaid fraud takes all forms. Patients who get and take what they aren't entitled to, and service providers who bill without providing services or for services different than provided. Fraud should not be tolerated in any form. I will work closely with our Rockland County District Attorney, Tom Zugibe, on these issues of fraud. More prosecutions will both punish the criminals and deter others from becoming criminals!

Figure 3   Political Officials Target Non-Beneficiaries with Messages about Medicaid

Source: www.barrykantrowitz.com/medicaid.html.

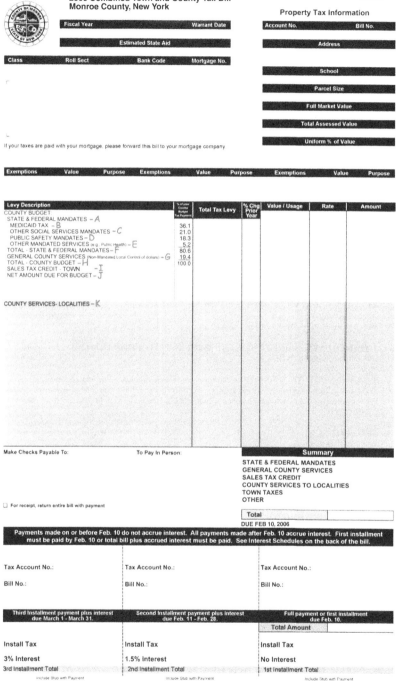

Figure 4 Example of a Tax Bill That Pinpoints Medicaid

LEVY DESCRIPTIONS
ON MONROE COUNTY TOWN AND COUNTY TAX BILL

<u>COUNTY BUDGET:</u>

A **STATE & FEDERAL MANDATES** are services that the County is either required to provide under State/Federal Law or State/Federal government funding requires these services to be provided.

    B **Medicaid Tax** funds an entitlement program that provides the cost of medical services for the elderly, disabled, and qualifying children & adults.

    C **Other Social Services Mandates** are programs which include Foster Care, Day Care, Safety Net, Family Assistance, Special Children's Services, Youth Bureau services, Office for the Aging Services, and Mental Health Services.

    D **Public Safety Mandates** are included in the following departments: Public Safety, Sheriff, District Attorney (DA), and Public Defender (PD). Some of the services include all of the DA & PD offices, Unified Court System, Probation, County Jail, Civil Bureau of the Sheriff's Office, and Court Security.

    E **Other Mandated Services** include State/Federal Mandates exclusive of the Social Services and Public Safety Mandates identified above. Some of the services include Monroe Community College as well as services provided by the Public Health Department.

F **TOTAL STATE & FEDERAL MANDATES** is the total of the County budget items listed above.

G **GENERAL COUNTY SERVICES** are the additional services provided by the County exclusive of those required by State/Federal Law. Some of the services include Sheriff's road patrol, County roads and bridges, County Parks, 911 Communication Center, and staff departments.

H **TOTAL COUNTY BUDGET** is the sum of the TOTAL STATE/FEDERAL MANDATES and the GENERAL COUNTY SERVICES.

I **SALES TAX CREDIT – (Town)** represents the share of total sales tax collections credited to towns (outside of villages). Whereas villages and the City of Rochester receive their total allocation of sales tax in cash, property owners in towns receive a portion of their sales tax as a credit, which reduces their property tax bill.

J **NET AMOUNT DUE FOR BUDGET** is equal to the TOTAL COUNTY BUDGET line less the SALES TAX CREDIT amount.

K **COUNTY SERVICES – LOCALITIES** consist of charges for Mutual Aid Fire Training, Election Expenses, Tax Roll and Bill Preparation, etc. which, under State Law, may be charged back to specific municipalities through assessments against property in those municipalities.

Figure 4 (Continued)

with policy confer lessons about government and politics. The PCF points to learning opportunities that extend beyond policy beneficiaries to the various groups of people living alongside them.

To be clear, the PCF details a wide range of relationships and social dynamics that I cannot fully explore in this article. It is an initial spring-board for theorizing concentration effects, but it is presently quite indefinite. Notice that I do not hypothesize about the *direction* of behavioral effects across contact types. On the one hand, social science research does not yet offer the theoretical tools necessary for understanding the range of ways that policy concentration will affect community members with different degrees of personal/direct contact. On the other hand, such effects are likely conditional and thus not easily pinpointed. For example, whether impersonal direct contact will mobilize, demobilize, or have no effect at all will depend on the nature of such contact (e.g., as a school nurse who sees students perform better when they have health coverage or as an overworked bureaucrat in an agency unsustainably serving more and more people). Similarly, while Hannah Walker (2014) shows that proximate contact (which I classify as personal and indirect) mobilizes, she also finds that the strength of this effect varies across racial groups. Though the same may hold true for Medicaid, it is also possible that indirect contact demobilizes in the domain of health where policy may be injurious, but it is not so punitive as to stoke a deep sense of social (in)justice.

All of this is to say that while the PCF serves as a basis for more precise hypothesizing in future research, this article cannot closely trace all of the paths that it illuminates. In fact, the aggregate data that I draw on does not allow me to distinguish types of policy contact. So, while the PCF establishes a basis for understanding *how* policy concentration might affect communities (i.e., mechanisms), the main task of this article is to garner initial evidence that it does so at all (i.e., effects).

A Focus on Counties

To decipher the effect of Medicaid density on local political participation, I examine county-level patterns. Aggregate county data provide ample geographic variation as well as some variation across time. Such data are sufficiently granular that they approximate (albeit imperfectly) community processes. At the same time, because counties are large and bear a significant responsibility for administering social programs, the government collects data on county-level Medicaid enrollment (this is not the case for neighborhoods or census tracts). For these reasons, county data are the best practical choice.

Counties also have more substantive significance. They represent "loci of government" capacity with measurable consequences for poverty, inequality, and governance (Benton 2002; Lobao et al. 2012; Sharp 2012). Counties are often the most proximate sites at which Medicaid benefits are administered. Though there is variation in the capacity of counties to make choices about the social programs they administer, the local caseworkers that they employ, train, and manage retain a tremendous amount of discretion (Sharp 2012: 31; Soss, Fording, and Schram 2011; Watkins-Hayes 2009). In addition, county Medicaid offices are sometimes located in visible places, where beneficiaries and non-beneficiaries alike can detect upsurges in enrollment and can develop ideas about which populations Medicaid serves. Finally, counties hold large enough numbers of people that they can facilitate not only the strong ties that characterize relationships with those most proximate to us, but also the weak ties that are useful for generating social and political capital (Granovetter 1973; Small 2009). Evidence suggests that counties are an important source of networks and social capital (Dillion 2011; Rupasingha, Goetz, and Freshwater 2006). This makes them a suitable context given the wide range of social relationships implicated in the PCF.

Data and Variables

The ensuing analyses are based on two key dependent variables. The first measures aggregate rates of voting in US counties during the 2000, 2004, and 2008 presidential elections. These data are drawn from CQ Press Voting and Elections Collection. Voting is a political outcome of central importance and it is frequently studied by social scientists. It is a basic act of democratic citizenship and is thus essential for the purpose of evaluating the political wherewithal of individuals and communities.

Still, voting is only one among a number of forms of participation. The second dependent variable measures another: the number of civic and political organizations in a given county each year between 2005 and 2010. These data come from the Census Bureau's County Business Patterns (CBP) Survey.[9] The associational life of communities is a vital marker of residents' capacity to mobilize politically (Kawachi, Venkata Subramanian, and Kim 2008; Putnam 2000).

Note that due to the time periods covered by the dependent variables, this research does not speak to the effect of the recent Medicaid expansion that has happened in the wake of the ACA. So, in contrast to Haselswerdt (2017) and Clinton and Sances (2017), I investigate the effect of *Medicaid concentration*, not expansion. These are quite distinct, as the former emphasizes the relevance of the distribution of Medicaid beneficiaries while the latter attends more generally to broadened access to the program. Naturally, the two are connected. Medicaid enrollment grows after an expansion, which affects patterns of concentration. Nevertheless,

___

9. Counts of civic and political associations were generated via the NAICS codes 813410 and 813940. These codes reflect the CBP data counts of the number of civic and political establishments (i.e., single physical locations) per county.

Medicaid concentration is a separate phenomenon that stems from a contextually contingent amalgam of race, class, and poverty governance. Admittedly, by investigating a period that does not include the most recent expansion of Medicaid, I lose the ability to examine how the political effects of concentration vary across different expansion/access regimes. I acknowledge that scope condition. One consolation is that the post-expansion period has been idiosyncratically marked by a large influx of new beneficiaries, ever-changing policy contours (with proliferating Section 1115 waivers), and a bitterly contentious national political scene. Interpreting patterns observed during this period would be challenging. Focusing on a pre-expansion time frame allows us to understand what happens during more stable times, when beneficiaries, bureaucrats, and policy makers are settled into comparatively routine and predictable patterns. Still, when data are available, scholars should also study the post-expansion period to assess whether and how the findings from the analyses below are altered by expansion.

Independent Variables

The primary independent variable in the models gauges Medicaid policy concentration by measuring the percent of county residents younger than 18 years old enrolled in Medicaid in a given year. These data come from the American Community Survey (ACS) and the Medicaid Statistical Information System (MSIS).[10] Since the percent of Medicaid beneficiaries under 18 years old is higher than the percent of adult beneficiaries, this variable represents the high bar for capturing how many people in a county have direct contact (even if on behalf of their children) with Medicaid. Moreover, in counties where high proportions of children are enrolled, community members who may never enroll in Medicaid (e.g., school administrators, nurses, etc.) can still encounter the program through exposure to its most common subpopulation: children. As suggested by the PCF, these direct impersonal contacts may be one mechanism through which program density has the potential to influence non-beneficiaries.

In addition to the variables described above, the analyses include controls for important time-varying demographic factors including population size, race (percent black and percent Hispanic), poverty, and income.

10. The actual Medicaid data used in the article were calculated by Sarah Miller (an economist at the University of Michigan), who generously shared her county-level Medicaid calculations with me. Miller mapped PUMA-level Medicaid enrollment rates from the ACS to the county level. For years prior to 2008, when ACS data were not available, Miller used state-level Medicaid enrollment data from MSIS to extrapolate county-level rates.

Table 3 Medicaid Concentration and Political Participation

	(1) Voting	(2) Associations
Child Medicaid density	–0.0709***	–0.119**
	(0.0165)	(0.0512)
Poverty (percentile)	0.00425***	0.00319**
	(0.000472)	(0.00145)
Median income	1.19e-06***	4.01e-06***
	(2.57e-07)	(1.06e-06)
Black	–0.0491	0.227
	(0.121)	(0.495)
Hispanic	–0.345***	–0.644
	(0.0490)	(0.510)
Population	1.45e-07***	–1.10e-07
	(3.92e-08)	(1.00e-07)
Observations (county-year)	8,944	16,027
County N	2,983	2,674

Note: Model 1 estimated using OLS Regression, Model 2 estimated *Poisson regression*. *Includes county fixed effects and year fixed effects* (not reported). Robust standard errors (in parentheses).
* $p < 0.1$, ** $p < 0.05$, *** $p < 0.01$

Analyses and Findings

The data used here contain information on over 2,600 counties. The voting models span three presidential elections (2000, 2004, and 2008), and the associational models track the presence of membership associations between 2005 and 2010. The unit of analysis is the county-year. Given relatively short time frames across many counties (small T, large N), I estimated panel regression models with county and year fixed effects (Cameron and Trivedi 2009). The first model predicts voting rates using an OLS estimator. The second model predicts counts of associations using a Poisson estimator.[11] All models are based on cluster robust

11. There are two relevant estimation techniques that I did not pursue. First, I considered using a negative binomial estimator for model 2 because the variance of outcome (count of associations) was large relative to its mean. However, the negative binomial model would not converge despite numerous attempts. Moreover, though Cameron and Trivedi (2009) suggest that Negative Binomial models can lead to improved efficiency, the Poisson panel estimators have the benefit of relying on weaker distributional assumptions, and may therefore be more robust given the use of cluster-robust standard errors (p. 641). A second issue is that over 400 counties were dropped from the Poisson model because they did not have any civic or political associations over the time period in question. To address this, I considered estimating a zero-inflated Poisson model. However, such models are inappropriate because they require that certain cases never be at risk of an event occurring.

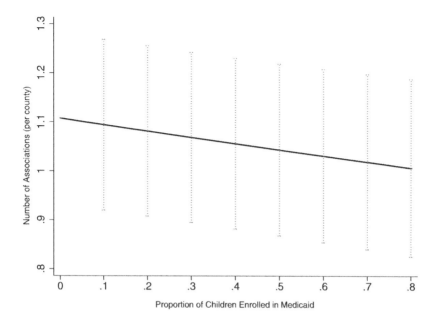

Figure 5 Medicaid Density and Local Associations

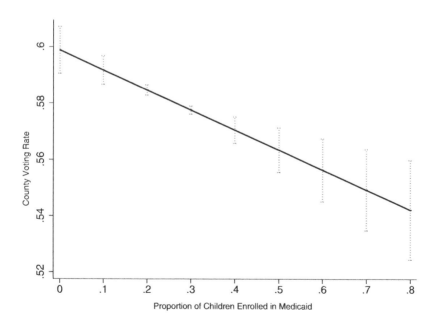

Figure 6 Medicaid Density and County Voting Rates

standard errors to account for heteroscedasticity and serial correlation (Cameron and Miller 2011).

Table 3 contains the main results. Model 1 provides evidence that child Medicaid density has a negative relationship to aggregate voting rates, and model 2 demonstrates a similarly negative correlation with the presence of civic and political membership associations in a county. Substantively, the significant negative coefficient on the Medicaid density variable in model 1 indicates that, for a given county, a 1 percent increase in child Medicaid enrollment (over time) is associated with a 7 percent decrease in county voting rates and an 11 percent decrease in the mean count of civic and political associations ($[e^{-.119}] - 1 = -.11$). These substantive effects are graphically depicted in figs. 5 and 6. The results support the hypothesis that Medicaid policy concentration is consequential for the political life of communities. Between 2000 and 2010, increasing rates of Medicaid enrollment had a dampening effect on local political participation.

Robustness of Findings

These findings warrant further empirical investigation. Four potential inferential challenges are especially obvious: (1) omitted variable bias, (2) conditional effects, (3) ecological fallacy, and (4) reverse causation. I'll discuss each in turn.

Omitted Variables

Though the use of fixed effects regression attenuates some concerns about omitted variable bias, the possibility of unaccounted for time-varying confounders remains. I cannot resolve this using observational data. However, I find reassuring indications in the results of models that I estimated including controls for unemployment, health (the incidence of premature death), and county-level political culture (percent voting Republican). Controlling for such factors does not alter the core findings.

One especially worrisome confounder is poverty. If Medicaid concentration is largely a stand-in for poverty (the bivariate correlation between these variables is 0.62), then its significance simply reflects the relationship between socioeconomic status and political participation. I take several steps to account for this possibility. First, I control for the percent of people who are below the poverty line in each county (see table 3). Doing so does not eliminate the statistical or substantive significance of the relationship

Table 4 Low Poverty Counties and Interactions (Robustness Tests)

	(1) Vote (Low-Poverty)	(2) Association (Low-Poverty)	(3) Vote (Interactions)
Child Medicaid density	−0.167***	−0.296*	−0.202***
	(0.0476)	(0.163)	(0.019)
Median income	7.91e-07**	4.49e-06**	1.04e-06***
	(3.85e-07)	(1.81e-06)	(2.47e-07)
Black	0.411***	−2.096	−0.277**
	(0.0918)	(1.655)	(0.117)
Hispanic	−0.417***	−0.594	−0.373***
	(0.109)	(1.504)	(0.050)
Population	1.91e-07***	1.50e-07	1.40e-07***
	(6.90e-08)	(4.84e-07)	(3.68e-08)
Poverty			0.003***
			(.000)
Black* child Medicaid			0.759***
density			(0.0506)
Rural* child Medicaid			−0.055***
density			(0.0204)
Observations	2,146	2,681	8,944
County *N*	990	576	2,983

Note: Models 1 and 3 estimated using OLS Regression, Model 2 estimated *Poisson regression*. *Includes county fixed effects and year fixed effects* (not reported). Robust standard errors (in parentheses).
* $p < 0.1$, ** $p < 0.05$, *** $p < 0.01$

between Medicaid concentration and either of the political outcomes. In fact, the substantive results are similar with or without controlling for poverty.

Making further efforts to address the entanglement of poverty and Medicaid concentration, I subset the data to include only low-poverty counties. The average poverty rate across all of the counties in the data set was 14 percent and the maximum was 54 percent. There were roughly 990 low-poverty counties (where fewer than 10 percent of residents were below the poverty line). Despite the comparatively minimal prevalence of poverty in these counties, there was still variation in child Medicaid enrollment. If confounded processes unique to poor counties are driving my results, then Medicaid concentration should not affect political participation in low-poverty counties. The subsetted models suggest the opposite (table 4, columns 1–2). The relationship between Medicaid density and political outcomes is significant and substantial in magnitude when the analyses are limited to places that are economically healthy relative to the rest of the country.

Conditional Relationships

Also relevant is whether the effect of Medicaid concentration is conditional on other factors. Most prominent among potential interactions are race, rural status, and the foreign-born composition of the county. Levels of Medicaid enrollment signal different things in different places, and the lens through which community members interpret the policy landscape may depend on the characteristics of the beneficiaries and the community members. In small rural towns where people know and trust one another, Medicaid may not carry the same stigma and Medicaid density may not exert the same dampening effect on participation (Michener forthcoming). Contrastingly, in places where a significant percent of the population is black or foreign-born, Medicaid density may prove especially demobilizing.

Also worth considering is the level of access that county residents have to doctors. Perhaps in counties where there is a shortage of doctors, Medicaid beneficiaries have negative (and potentially demobilizing) experiences stemming from their inability to access care. Further still, is the possibility that in these places non-beneficiaries also lack access, making it more likely that they will view Medicaid beneficiaries negatively or blame them for overburdening the health care system. Either way, doctor shortages could be an additional factor conditioning the effect of Medicaid concentration.

An analysis of interactions suggests that some of these factors are important, but not all. The (negative) correlation between Medicaid concentration and county-level voting rates increases (i.e., there is a positive and significant interaction) as the black share of the population increases (see table 4, column 3). The opposite holds for rural status: the relationship between voting and Medicaid concentration is attenuated in counties that are designated as rural (a negative and significant interaction). However, the effects of Medicaid concentration are not conditional on the proportion of county residents who are foreign-born or on whether a county is designated as a primary care health professional shortage area (insignificant interactions not shown). Furthermore, none of the conditional effects hold for the associational models.

Ecological Fallacy

The findings presented above are based on aggregate analyses of county-level data and thus do not give us much leverage for making inferences about the political behavior of individuals. Yet, the mechanisms by which county voting rates and associational activity decline in response to Medicaid density necessarily involve individual political action. Prior studies referenced earlier consider the influence of Medicaid enrollment on the political behavior of individuals (Michener, forthcoming), but not the influence of Medicaid density (a contextual factor) on such behavior. Evidence that Medicaid density has an influence on individual-level political outcomes (net of the influence of individual-level Medicaid enrollment) would support the argument that the effects of policy concentration are distinct.

To assess individual-level patterns, I turn to the third wave of the Fragile Families and Child Well-Being Study (FFS). This survey follows a cohort of nearly 5,000 children born in US cities, interviewing both mothers and fathers around the time of their child's birth and at various intervals subsequently. Since the sample was composed to reflect non-marital births in large US cities, it is not nationally representative in the traditional sense. However, the emphasis on "fragile families" means that FFS contains an unusually large number of poor persons. These data are uniquely well suited for studying low-income populations (Bruch, Marx Ferree, and Soss 2010). Questions about political activity were only asked in the third wave (2001/2004), so that cross-section is employed here. There were 7,529 respondents interviewed in wave three (with an average response rate of 77 percent). Among this number, 53 percent (just under 4,000 persons) reported that either they or their children were enrolled in Medicaid, providing uncommon empirical leverage for understanding patterns of political behavior.[12]

To generate a Medicaid density variable, I aggregated at the census tract level (the lowest level for which FFS has a geographic identifier). This is not ideal, because there are 2,100 census tracts and the number of respondents in many tracts is quite small. This limitation notwithstanding, I estimate a set of models aimed at gauging whether tract-level Medicaid density is significantly correlated with political and civic outcomes, net of numerous other factors.

To confront some of the challenges that accompany cross-sectional observational analyses, I use robust standard errors clustered at the census tract level. I also use a quasi-experimental *matching* technique to ensure that the effect of individual-level Medicaid enrollment is accounted for as

---

12. Notably, Medicaid beneficiaries in the FFS sample are not reflective of the Medicaid population nationally; FFS beneficiaries are younger, healthier, more likely to be male, and less likely to live below the poverty line.

best as possible (Iacus et al. 2012).[13] Matching addresses the confounding influence of factors causally prior to the primary independent variable by better aligning the distributions of observed covariates in the treatment group (Medicaid beneficiaries) with those in the control group (non-beneficiaries). This technique (imperfectly) approximates the counter-factual condition where those being studied are similar in every way except for Medicaid participation. Estimates produced by using matched data are less sensitive to model specification, less biased, and more efficient (Ho et al. 2007).[14]

Using data pre-processed via the matching procedure, I estimate voter registration and civic attitudes.[15] Drawing on insights from the political participation literature, I control for key individual characteristics including age, education, employment, income, sex, race, nativity, cash welfare receipt, and church attendance (Rosenstone and Hansen 1993; Verba et al. 1995). I also include a control for self-rated health and controls at the census tract level for race (percent black and Hispanic, respectively) and poverty (percent below the poverty line). The models predict each political outcome as a function of individual-level Medicaid enrollment, census tract level Medicaid density and all of the controls. The voter turnout and registration models were estimated via probit and the broader participation model (which includes being part of a political group and attending a rally) via ordinary least squares.

As shown in table 5, Medicaid density is significantly and negatively correlated with voting and political participation. These results should be interpreted cautiously. They are based on self-reported voting and cross-sectional analysis, which comes with a host of inferential challenges that matching and clustered errors do not solve. Medicaid enrollment at the individual level and Medicaid density are highly correlated ($\alpha = .71$), so the non-significance of the individual-level Medicaid variable in this model should not be taken to mean that the individual experiences do not matter,

13. Coarsened exact matching is a multi-step process: (1) temporarily coarsen X (i.e., recode it to assume fewer values), (2) perform exact matching on the coarsened X by sorting observations into strata with unique values of C(X), (3) eliminate any stratum missing treatment or control variables, (4) pass on original uncoarsened variables, except those omitted as per step #3, and (5) analyze original data using stratum derived from step #2 as weights in the analysis.

14. The variables used in the matching procedure were: age, sex, TANF participation, education, race (black), marital status, and household income. I selected covariates likely to influence both the treatment and outcomes, while omitting variables that could be affected by the treatment (e.g., health), and thus induce post-treatment bias.

15. Civic attitudes were measured using a scale combining respondents' ratings of the importance of five activities: voting, serving in the military, jury duty, volunteering, and reporting a crime. Relatively few respondents were part of a community group or political group, so I opted to use an attitudinal measure of civic capacity, which is a likely mechanism for the associational outcome observed in the aggregate data.

Table 5 Medicaid Density and Individual Attitudes/Behavior

	(1) Vote	(2) Register	(3) Political Participation
Individual Level Variables			
Medicaid	0.144	−0.183**	0.0231
	(0.0952)	(0.0907)	(0.0321)
Age	0.0206***	0.00903*	0.00867***
	(0.00597)	(0.00545)	(0.00216)
Sex	−0.180**	−0.0882	−0.0325
	(0.0732)	(0.0644)	(0.0262)
Employed	0.00596	−0.236***	−0.0660***
	(0.0701)	(0.0660)	(0.0233)
Health	−0.0167	0.0487*	0.0167
	(0.0317)	(0.0273)	(0.0117)
US Born	−0.0860	−1.592***	−0.328***
	(0.156)	(0.0946)	(0.0430)
Income	0.0205	0.0312	0.0262
	(0.0552)	(0.0521)	(0.0238)
Poverty (percentile)	0.0949**	0.0362	0.0280
	(0.0438)	(0.0338)	(0.0178)
TANF	0.148	−0.442	−0.0377
	(0.192)	(0.294)	(0.0661)
Education	0.222***	0.289***	0.138***
	(0.0442)	(0.0377)	(0.0152)
Black	0.157*	0.176**	0.0840**
	(0.0949)	(0.0879)	(0.0343)
Latino	−0.128	0.116	0.00450
	(0.0906)	(0.0814)	(0.0339)
Church	−0.0511**	−0.0471**	−0.0297***
	(0.0206)	(0.0196)	(0.00777)
Civic attitude	0.112***	0.0884***	0.0452***
	(0.0189)	(0.0182)	(0.00624)
Tract Level Variables			
Medicaid (tract density)	−0.337**	0.151	-.094*
	(0.135)	(0.126)	(0.050)
Black			0.125***
	0.386**	0.272**	(.046)
	(0.123)	(0.117)	
Poverty	0.250	0.558**	0.245**
	(0.284)	(0.274)	(0.104)
N	3,706	5,213	5,234

especially given the low numbers of Medicaid beneficiaries in some tracts. The larger point here is to provide prima facie evidence that individual-level patterns correspond to aggregate outcomes observed in the county-level data. To that end, it is especially instructive to observe that the relationships are negative, and that they apply to outcomes that map on to those measured in the aggregate analyses.

Reverse Causation

Another important consideration is reverse or reciprocal causation. Research suggests that civically and politically active communities attract greater resources and do a better job of disseminating health information (Viswanath, Randolph Steele, and Finnegan 2006). If such communities facilitate better health, then residents may have lower demand for Medicaid. In essence, politically engaged counties may have a smaller proportion of residents enrolled in Medicaid because the benefits of living in such places dampen the need for Medicaid.

There are several reasons why this causal interpretation is not convincing. Even in communities that attract health resources (clinics, hospitals), health insurance remains indispensable and such resources should enable residents to have greater access to health coverage (health-related institutions often assist with enrollment in Medicaid). In addition, communities with the means for disseminating health information are also best equipped to spread the word about Medicaid to uninsured or needy residents (Viswanath, Randolph Steele, and Finnegan 2006). By this logic, the benefits of political participation should increase Medicaid enrollment in civic-minded communities (*ceteris paribus*). If politically engaged communities influence Medicaid enrollment rates, they should do so in a positive direction. The finding of a negative relationship between Medicaid density and political participation suggests that different processes are at work.

Policy Implications

The 1970s and 1980s ushered in a shift of national anti-poverty policy away from place-based strategies targeting disadvantaged locales and toward people-based policies that provide resources to individuals without regard to where they live (Kincaid 1999, 2012; O'Connor 1999; Partridge and Rickman 2006; Rich 1993). Despite retrenchment on the front of traditional cash assistance (Aid to Families with Dependent Children/Temporary Assistance for Needy Families), in-kind, people-based policies such as the Women, Infants and Children Nutrition Program (WIC) and the

Supplemental Nutrition Assistance Program (SNAP) have enrolled growing numbers of individuals since the 1970s (Moffitt 2015). Moreover, tax-based policies such as the Earned Income Tax Credit (EITC) have also expanded substantially during this time. Finally, Medicaid has grown exponentially, emerging (both fiscally and in terms of enrollment) as chief among people-based, means-tested policies. Most crucially, during the very same time period that Medicaid and the other programs cited above have been swelling, streams of funds dedicated to the needs of local communities have dried up. For instance, in 1978 approximately 15 percent of city revenues came from federal aid; today that number ranges from 1 to 3 percent (Kincaid 1999). Between 1980 and 1990, the Reagan and Bush administrations slashed grants to cities by 46 percent (Katz 1995). Community Development Block Grants were cut by 25 percent, urban jobs programs disappeared and General Revenue Sharing, which had previously provided localities with some funding, was eliminated (Katz 1995; Kincaid 2011). Altogether, federal grants-in-aid to state and local governments for resources distributed directly to people have increased markedly since the mid-1970s, while outlays for programs aimed at places have plummeted (Kincaid 2012).

By offering evidence that Medicaid density is associated with county-level political demobilization, this research underscores the risks of such an exclusively people-based approach to reducing health disparities and other inequities. If politically empowering communities with vulnerable health care constituents facilitates achieving health equity (as I argue it does), then policies that offer people access to health resources must not simultaneously weaken the political strength of their communities. Instead, the distinct geography of disadvantage in the United States necessitates that policies are responsive to both people *and* places.

This is possible if we complement Medicaid's people-based design with additional resources directed to the most needy communities. Specific efforts might include increasing the funding for and capacity of Community Health Centers, subsidizing community-based health initiatives, and offering greater support for civic and political organizations in distressed communities.[16] This also provides a reason to consider the kinds of direct action that government can take to empower the beneficiaries of people-based policies. Though the feasibility of this recommendation is highly contingent on political climate, one promising route would be for the federal government and states to ensure full cooperation with the National

---

16. For an example of what the CDC under the Obama administration has done on this: www.cdc.gov/nccdphp/dch/programs/partnershipstoimprovecommunityhealth/index.html.

Voter Registration Act, particularly Section 7. This statute mandates that public assistance agencies offer every applicant and enrollee an opportunity to register to vote. Recent research indicates that compliance with Section 7 is lax in many states, especially those with growing numbers of black Americans (Michener 2016). Shoring up this law and applying it more equitably is a step toward offsetting the potentially demobilizing community-level repercussions of people-based policies such as Medicaid. Similarly, any local political activity that reinforces the political incorporation of social policy beneficiaries may be useful in this regard (e.g., organizing political meetings or voter registration drives at local health facilities).

Additionally, foundations with resources to fund grassroots organizations (and those organizations themselves) should be mindful of these patterns when deciding which communities to serve, and should consider cultivating political capital in places where community-wide experiences with policy might otherwise erode it. Policy makers, community planners, and other key players must be cognizant of how places shape the political impact of social policy. Attentiveness to collective political capital should be part of policy discourse and should inform strategies to alleviate health (and other) disparities.

Finally, local political elites who sometimes use Medicaid and other public assistance programs as fodder for their own political ends should closely consider the potential democratic consequences of their actions. Stigmatizing Medicaid (especially in places where many people rely on it) has downstream consequences for how beneficiaries, their family members, and their neighbors think about and engage in politics. While we still have much to learn about the processes through which this happens, this work suggests that the local-level understandings of such programs may have significant stakes. Those who set the terms of political discourse must attend to this possibility.

■ ■ ■

Jamila D. Michener is an assistant professor of Government at Cornell University. She studies the politics of poverty, racial inequality, and public policy in the United States. Her research has been published in several book chapters and numerous journals, including the journals *Political Behavior, Poverty and Public Policy* and *The Forum*. Her book (forthcoming with Cambridge University Press) examines how Medicaid—a pillar of the US welfare state and a paragon of federalism—affects political life in economically and racially marginalized communities.
jm2362@cornell.edu

Acknowledgments

I would like to thank the participants of the Robert Wood Johnson Investigators Awards Annual Meeting (September 2016), as well as participants in the City and Regional Planning graduate seminar (November 2016) for their invaluable feedback. I am particularly indebted to Suzanne Mettler, Julia Lynch, Leslie Hinkson, Keith Wailoo, and the editors of this issue.

References

Acevedo-Garcia, Dolores, and Kimberly A. Lochner. 2003. "Residential Segregation and Health." In *Neighborhoods and Health*, edited by Ichiro Kawachi and Lisa F. Berkman, 265–87. New York: Oxford University Press.

Alex-Assensoh, Yvette. 1997. "Race, Concentrated Poverty, Social Isolation, and Political Behavior." *Urban Affairs Review* 33, no. 2: 209–27.

Andrews, Christina. 2014. "Unintended Consequences: Medicaid Expansion and Racial Inequality in Access to Health Insurance." *Health and Social Work* 39, no. 3: 131–33.

Auchincloss, Amy H., and Wilbur Hadden. 2002. "The Health Effects of Rural-Urban Residence and Concentrated Poverty." *Journal of Rural Health* 18, no. 2: 319–36.

Baicker, Katherine, Sarah L. Taubman, Heidi Allen, Mira Bernstein, Johnathan Gruber, Joseph Newhouse, Efrain Schneider, Bill J. Wright, Alan M. Zaslavsky, and Amy N Finkelstein. 2013. "The Oregon Experiment—Effects of Medicaid on Clinical Outcomes." *New England Journal of Medicine* 368: 1713–22.

Bambra, Clare, Debbie Fox, and Alex Scott-Samuel. 2005. "Towards a Politics of Health." *Health Promotion International* 20, no. 2: 187–93.

Benton, Edwin J. 2002. *Counties as Service Delivery Agents: Changing Expectations and Roles*. Westport, CT: Praeger.

Browning, Christopher R., and Kathleen A. Cagney. 2002. *Journal of Health and Social Behavior* 43, no. 4: 383–99.

Bruch, Sarah K., Myra Marx Ferree, and Joe Soss. 2010. "From Policy to Polity: Democracy, Paternalism, and the Incorporation of Disadvantaged Citizens." *American Sociological Review* 75, no. 2: 205–26.

Burch, Traci. 2013. *Trading Democracy for Justice: Criminal Convictions and the Decline of Neighborhood Participation*. Chicago: University of Chicago Press.

Cameron, A. Colin, and Pravin K. Trivedi. 2009. *Microeconometrics Using Stata*. College Station, TX: Stata.

Cameron, A. Colin, and Douglas L. Miller. 2011. "Robust Inference with Clustered Data." In *Handbook of Empirical Economics and Finance*, edited by A. Ullah and D. E. Giles, 1–28. Boca Raton, FL: CRC.

Campbell, Andrea Louise. 2003. *How Policies Make Citizens: Senior Political Activism and the American Welfare State*. Princeton, NJ: Princeton University Press.

Campbell, Andrea Louise. 2012. "Policy Makes Mass Politics." *Annual Review of Political Science* 15: 333–51.

Campbell, Andrea Louise. 2014. *Trapped in America's Safety Net: One Family's Struggle.* Chicago: University of Chicago Press.

Cattell, Vicky. 2001. "Poor People, Poor Places, and Poor Health: The Mediating Role of Social Networks and Social Capital." *Social Science and Medicine* 52, no. 10: 1501–16.

Chetty, Raj, Nathaniel Hendren, and Lawrence F. Katz. 2016. "The Effects of Exposure to Better Neighborhoods on Children: New Evidence from the Moving to Opportunity Experiment." *American Economic Review* 106, no. 4: 855–902.

Clinton, Joshua, and Michael A. Sances. 2017. "The Politics of Policy: The Initial Mass Political Effects of Medicaid Expansion in the States." Working Paper. http://csap.yale.edu/sites/default/files/files/apppw_jc_3-8-17_paper.pdf.

Cohen, Cathy J., and Michael C. Dawson. 1993. "Neighborhood Poverty and African-American Politics." *American Political Science Review* 87: 286–302.

Cohodes, Sarah R., Daniel S. Grossman, Samuel A. Kleiner, and Michael F. Lovenheim. 2014. "The Effect of Child Health Insurance Access on Schooling: Evidence from Public Insurance Expansions." *Journal of Human Resources* 51, no. 3: 727–59.

Dillon, Michele. 2011. "Stretching Ties: Social Capital and the Rebranding of Coös County, New Hampshire." Carsey Institute, New England Issues Brief No. 27.

Do, D. Phuong, Brian Karl Finch, Ricardo Basurto-Davila, Chloe Bird, Jose Escarce, and Nicole Lurie. 2008. "Does Place Explain Racial Health Disparities? Quantifying the Contribution of Residential Context to the Black/White Health Gap in the United States." *Social Science and Medicine* 67, no. 8: 1258–68.

Dreier, Peter, John H. Mollenkopf, and Todd Swanstrom. 2004. *Place Matters: Metropolitics for the Twenty-First Century.* Lawrence: University Press of Kansas.

Finch, Brian K., D. Phuong Do, Melonie Heron, Chloe Bird, Teresa Seeman, and Nicole Lurie. 2010. "Neighborhood Effects on Health: Concentrated Advantage and Disadvantage." *Health and Place* 16, no. 5: 1058–60.

Fiscella, Kevin, and David R. Williams. 2004. "Health Disparities Based on Socioeconomic Inequities: Implications for Urban Health Care." *Academic Medicine* 79, no. 12: 1139–47.

Gaskin, Darrell J., Roland J. Thorpe Jr., Emma E. McGinty, Kelly Bower, Charles Rohde, J. Hunter Young, Thomas A. LaVeist, and Lisa Dubay. 2014. "Disparities in Diabetes: The Nexus of Race, Poverty, and Place." *American Journal of Public Health* 104, no. 11: 2147–55.

Grady, Sue C. 2006. "Racial Disparities in Low Birthweight and the Contribution of Residential Segregation: A Multilevel Analysis." *Social Science and Medicine* 63, no. 12: 3013–29.

Granovetter, Mark S. 1973. "The Strength of Weak Ties." *American Journal of Sociology* 78, no. 6: 1360–80.

Han, Hahrie. 2009. *Moved to Action: Motivation, Participation, and Inequality in American Politics.* Stanford: Stanford University Press.

Haselswerdt, Jake. 2017. "Expanding Medicaid, Expanding the Electorate: The Affordable Care Act's Short-Term Impact on Political Participation." *Journal of Health Politics, Policy and Law* 42, no. 4: 667–95.

Ho, Daniel E., Kosuke Imai, Gary King, and Elizabeth A. Stuart. 2007. "Matching as Nonparametric Preprocessing for Reducing Model Dependence in Parametric Causal Inference." *Political Analysis* 15, no. 3: 199–236.

Iacus, Stefano M., Gary King, Giuseppe Porro, and Jonathan N. Katz. 2012. "Causal Inference Without Balance Checking: Coarsened Exact Matching." *Political Analysis* 20, no. 1: 1–24.

Jacob, Brian A., Jens Ludwig, and Douglas L. Miller. 2013. "The Effects of Housing and Neighborhood Conditions on Child Mortality." *Journal of Health Economics* 32, no. 1: 195–206.

Jargowsky, Paul. 2015. *The Architecture of Segregation: Civil Unrest, the Concentration of Poverty and Public Policy.* New York: Century Foundation.

Katz, Michael B. 1995. *Improving Poor People: The Welfare State, The "Underclass," and Urban Schools as History.* Princeton, NJ: Princeton University Press.

Kawachi, Ichiro, Sankaran Venkata Subramanian, and Daniel Kim. 2008. "Social Capital and Health." In *Social Capital and Health,* edited by Ichiro Kawachi, Sankaran Venkata Subramanian and Daniel Kim, 1–26. New York: Springer.

Kincaid, John. 1999. "De Facto Devolution and Urban Defunding: The Priority of Persons over Places." *Journal of Urban Affairs* 21: 135–67.

Kincaid, John. 2012. "The Rise of Social Welfare and Onward March of Coercive Federalism." In *Networked Governance: The Future of Intergovernmental Management,* edited by Jack W. Meek and Kurt Thurmaier, 8–33. Washington, DC: CQ.

Kneebone, Elizabeth, and Carey Ann Nadeau. 2015. "The Resurgence on Concentrated Poverty in America: Metropolitan Trends in the 2000s." In *The New American Suburb: Poverty, Race and the Economic Crisis,* edited by K. B. Anacker, 15–38. New York: Routledge.

Krivo, Lauren J., Ruth D. Peterson, Helen Rizzo, and John R. Reynolds. 1998. "Race, Segregation, and the Concentration of Disadvantage: 1980–1990." *Social Problems* 45, no. 1: 61–80.

LaVeist, Thomas A. 1989. "Linking Residential Segregation and the Infant Mortality Race Disparity." *Sociology and Social Research* 73, no. 2: 90–94.

LaVeist, Thomas A. 1992. "The Political Empowerment and Health Status of African-Americans: Mapping a New Territory." *American Journal of Sociology* 97, no. 4: 1080–95.

Lerman, Amy, and Vesla Weaver. 2014. *Arresting Citizenship: The Democratic Consequences of American Crime Control.* Chicago: University of Chicago Press.

Levitsky, Sandra R. 2014. *Caring for Our Own: Why There Is No Political Demand for New American Social Welfare Rights.* New York: Oxford University Press.

Lobao, Linda, P., Wilner Jeanty, Mark Partridge, and David Kraybill. 2012. "Poverty and Place across the United States: Do County Governments Matter to the Distribution of Economic Disparities?" *International Regional Science Review* 35, no. 2: 158–87.

Ludwig, Jens, Greg J. Duncan, Lisa A. Gennetian, Lawrence F. Katz, Ronald C. Kessler, Jeffrey R. Kling, and Lisa Sanbonmatsu. 2013. "Long-Term Neighborhood Effects on Low-Income Families: Evidence from Moving to Opportunity." *American Economic Review* 103, no. 3: 226–31.

Lukens, Gideon. 2014. "State Variation in Health Care Spending and the Politics of State Medicaid Policy." *Journal of Health Politics, Policy and Law* 39, no. 6: 1213–51.

MacGillis, Alec. 2015. "Who Turned My Blue State Red? Why Poor Areas Vote for Politicians Who Want to Slash the Safety Net." *New York Times*, November 20.

Marcus, Andrea Fleisch, Sandra E. Echeverria, Bart K. Holland, Ana F. Abraido-Lanza, and Marian R. Passannante. 2016. "The Joint Contribution of Neighborhood Poverty and Social Integration to Mortality Risk in the United States." *Annals of Epidemiology* 26, no. 4: 261–66.

Massey, Douglas S., and Nancy Denton. 1993. *American Apartheid: Segregation and the Making of the Underclass.* Cambridge, MA: Harvard University Press.

Massey, Douglas S., and Kumiko Shibuya. 1995. "Unraveling the Tangle of Pathology: The Effect of Spatially Concentrated Joblessness on the Well-Being of African Americans." *Social Science Research* 24, no. 4: 352–66.

Mettler, Suzanne. 2005. *Soldiers to Citizens: The GI Bill and the Making of the Greatest Generation.* New York: Oxford University Press.

Mettler, Suzanne, and Joe Soss. 2004. "The Consequences of Public Policy for Democratic Citizenship: Bridging Policy Studies and Mass Politics." *Perspectives on Politics* 2 (March): 55–73.

Michener, Jamila. 2013. "Neighborhood Disorder and Local Participation: Examining the Political Relevance of 'Broken Windows.'" *Political Behavior* 35, no. 4: 777–806.

Michener, Jamila. 2016. "Race, Poverty, and the Redistribution of Voting Rights." *Poverty and Public Policy* 8, no. 2: 106–28.

Michener, Jamila. Forthcoming. *Fragmented Democracy: Medicaid, Federalism and Unequal Politics.* New York: Cambridge University Press.

Miller, Lisa L. 2008. *The Perils of Federalism: Race, Poverty and the Politics of Crime Control.* New York: Oxford University Press.

Moffitt, Robert A. 2015. "The Deserving Poor, the Family, and the U.S. Welfare System." *Demography* 52, no. 3: 729–49.

Navarro, Vicente, and Leiyu Shi. 2001. "The Political Context of Social Inequalities and Health." *Social Science and Medicine* 52, no. 3: 481–91.

Norton, Mira, Bianca DiJulio, and Mollyann Brodie. 2015. "Medicare and Medicaid at 50." Kaiser Family Foundation. http://kff.org/medicaid/poll-finding/medicare-and-medicaid-at-50/.

O'Connor, Alice. 1999. "Swimming against the Tide: A Brief History of Federal Policy in Poor Communities." In *Urban Problems and Community Development*, edited by R. F. Ferguson and W. T. Dickens, 77–137. Washington, DC: Brookings Institution.

Ohmer, Mary L. 2007. "Citizen Participation in Neighborhood Organizations and Its Relationship to Volunteers' Self- and Collective Efficacy and Sense of Community." *Social Work Research* 31, no. 2: 109–20.

Pacheco, Julianna, and Jason Fletcher. 2015. "Incorporating Health into Studies of Political Behavior: Evidence for Turnout and Partisanship." *Political Research Quarterly* 68, no. 1: 104–16.

Paradise, Julia. 2015. "Medicaid Moving Forward." Kaiser Family Foundation. http://kff.org/health-reform/issue-brief/medicaid-moving-forward/.

Partridge, M. D., and D. S. Rickman. 2006. *The Geography of American Poverty: Is There a Need for Place-Based Policies?* Kalamazoo, MI: W. E. Upjohn Institute.

Pierson, Paul. 1993. "When Effect Becomes Cause: Policy Feedback and Political Change." *World Politics* 45: 595–628.

Putnam, Robert D. 2000. *Bowling Alone: The Collapse and Revival of American Community*. New York: Simon and Schuster.

Rich, Michael J. 1993. *National Goals and Local Choices: Distributing Federal Aid to the Poor*. Princeton, NJ: Princeton University Press.

Rosenstone Steven J. and John Mark Hansen. 1993. *Mobilization, Participation, and Democracy in America*. New York: Macmillan.

Rothstein, Richard. 2014. *The Making of Ferguson: Public Policies at the Root of Its Troubles*. Washington, DC: Economic Policy Institute.

Rudowitz, Robin, Laura Snyder and Vernon K. Smith. 2015. "Medicaid Enrollment and Spending Growth: FY 2015 and 2016." Menlo Park: The Kaiser Commission on Medicaid and the Uninsured.

Rupasingha, Anil, Stephan J. Goetz, and David Freshwater. 2006. "The Production of Social Capital in US Counties." *Journal of Socio-Economics* 35, no. 1: 83–101.

Schlozman, Kay Lehman, Sidney Verba, and Henry E. Brady. 2012. *The Unheavenly Chorus: Unequal Political Voice and the Broken Promise of American Democracy*. Princeton: Princeton University Press.

Schneider, Anne, and Helen Ingram. 1993. "Social Construction of Target Populations: Implications for Politics and Policy." *American Political Science Review* 87, no. 2: 334–47.

Schroeder, Steven A. 2007. "We Can Do Better—Improving the Health of the American People." *New England Journal of Medicine* 357, no. 12: 1221–28.

Sharkey, Patrick. 2013. *Stuck in Place: Urban Neighborhoods and the End of Progress toward Racial Equality*. Chicago: University of Chicago Press.

Sharp, Elaine B. 2012. *Does Local Government Matter? How Urban Policies Shape Civic Engagement*. Minneapolis: University of Minnesota Press.

Skocpol, Theda. 1992. *Protecting Soldiers and Mothers: The Political Origins of Social Policy in the United States*. Cambridge, MA: Belknap Press.

Small, Mario Luis. 2009. *Unanticipated Gains: Origins of Network Inequality in Everyday Life*. New York: Oxford University Press.

Sommers, Benjamin, Katherine Baicker and Arnold Epstein. 2012. "Mortality and Access to Care among Adults after State Medicaid Expansions." *New England Journal of Medicine* 367: 1025–34.

Soroka, Stuart Neil, and Christopher. Wlezien. 2010. *Degrees of Democracy: Politics, Public Opinion, and Policy*. New York: Cambridge University Press.

Soss, Joe. 1999. "Lessons of Welfare: Policy Design, Political Learning, and Political Action." *American Political Science Review* 93, no. 2: 363–80.

Soss, Joe. 2000. *Unwanted Claims: The Politics of Participation in the U.S. Welfare System*. Ann Arbor: University of Michigan Press.

Soss, Joe, Richard C. Fording, and Sanford F. Schram. 2011. *Disciplining the Poor: Neoliberal Paternalism and the Persistent Power of Race*. Chicago: University of Chicago Press.

Soss, Joe and Sanford F. Schram. 2007. "A Public Transformed? Welfare Reform as Policy Feedback." *American Political Science Review* 101, no. 1: 111–27.

Sparer, Michael S. 1996. *Medicaid and the Limits of State Health Reform*. Philadelphia: Temple University Press.

Szreter, Simon, and Michael Woolcock. 2004. "Health by Association? Social Capital, Social Theory, and the Political Economy of Public Health." *International Journal of Epidemiology* 33: 650–67.

Verba, Sidney, Kay Lehman Schlozman, and Henry E. Brady. 1995. *Voice and Equality: Civic Voluntarism in American Politics*. Cambridge: Harvard University Press.

Viswanath, Kasisomayajula, Whitney Randolph Steele, and John R. Finnegan Jr. 2006. "Social Capital and Health: Civic Engagement, Community Size, and Recall of Health Messages." *American Journal of Public Health* 96, no. 8: 1456–61.

Wallerstein, Nina. 1992. "Powerlessness, Empowerment, and Health: Implications for Health Promotion Programs." *American Journal of Health Promotion* 6, no. 3: 197–205.

Walker, Hannah L. 2014. "Extending the Effects of the Carceral State: Proximal Contact, Political Participation, and Race." *Political Research Quarterly* 67, no. 4: 809–22.

Watkins-Hayes, Celeste. 2009. *The New Welfare Bureaucrats: Entanglements of Race, Class, and Policy Reform*. Chicago: University of Chicago Press.

Williams, David R., and Chiquita Collins. 2001. "Racial Residential Segregation: A Fundamental Cause of Racial Disparities in Health." *Public Health Reports* 116, no. 5: 404.

Wilson, William J. 1987. *The Truly Disadvantaged: The Inner City, the Underclass, and Public Policy*. Chicago: University of Chicago Press.

Wlezien, Christopher. "The Public as Thermostat: Dynamics of Preferences for Spending." *American Journal of Political Science* 1995: 981–1000.

Yen, Irene H., and George A. Kaplan. 1999. "Poverty Area Residence and Changes in Depression and Perceived Health Status: Evidence from the Alameda County Study." *International Journal of Epidemiology* 28, no. 1: 90–94.

Young, Jr., Alford. 2003. "Social Isolation, and Concentration Effects: William Julius Wilson Revisited and Re-applied." *Ethnic and Racial Studies* 26, no. 6: 1073–87.

Young, Frank W., and Nina Glasgow. 1998. "Voluntary Social Participation and Health." *Research on Aging* 20, no. 3: 339–62.

Missed Opportunity? Leveraging Mobile Technology to Reduce Racial Health Disparities

Rashawn Ray
University of Maryland

Abigail A. Sewell
Emory University

Keon L. Gilbert
Saint Louis University

Jennifer D. Roberts
University of Maryland

Abstract Blacks and Latinos are less likely than whites to access health insurance and utilize health care. One way to overcome some of these racial barriers to health equity may be through advances in technology that allow people to access and utilize health care in innovative ways. Yet, little research has focused on whether the racial gap that exists for health care utilization also exists for accessing health information online and through mobile technologies. Using data from the Health Information National Trends Survey (HINTS), we examine racial differences in obtaining health information online via mobile devices. We find that blacks and Latinos are more likely to trust online newspapers to get health information than whites. Minorities who have access to a mobile device are more likely to rely on the Internet for health information in a time of strong need. Federally insured individuals who are connected to mobile devices have the highest probability of reliance on the Internet as a go-to source of health information. We conclude by discussing the importance of mobile technologies for health policy, particularly related to developing health literacy, improving health outcomes, and contributing to reducing health disparities by race and health insurance status.

Keywords health disparities, race, minority health, mobile phone technology, health policy

Blacks and Latinos are more likely to live in poor neighborhoods, have higher rates of mortality, and suffer from chronic diseases (Gilbert et al. 2016; Gilbert, Ray, and Langston 2014; Massey and Denton 1993; Sewell

Funding for this project was provided by the Robert Wood Johnson Foundation Health Policy Research Program.

Journal of Health Politics, Policy and Law, Vol. 42, No. 5, October 2017
DOI 10.1215/03616878-3940477   © 2017 by Duke University Press

2010). Wealth and economic segregation is important when thinking about racial differences in health outcomes, considering that the high level of obesity among blacks is explained away by their likelihood of living in poverty (Boardman et al. 2005; Diez-Roux 2001, 2011; Hajat et al. 2010; Kawachi and Berkman 2003). As a result, scholars consider our racial residential segregation as a fundamental cause of health disparities (Kwate et al. 2009; Williams and Collins 1995).

In addition to housing segregation, blacks and Latinos face labor market discrimination that restricts their access from jobs that provide quality health insurance (Stainback and Tomaskovic-Devey 2012). Consequently, blacks and Latinos are less likely to utilize health care and face a daunting health insurance gap. As of 2014, nearly 30 percent of adults who are Latino or living in poverty, as well as over 15 percent of adult blacks, compared to around 10 percent of adult whites, did not have health insurance coverage.[1] Besides the insurance gap, blacks are less likely to trust physicians (Sewell 2015). Due to a lack of communication between minority patients and health care providers, compared to white patients, and the fact that health care personnel mistakenly perceive blacks as having higher pain thresholds, minorities often receive fewer services and lower quality care (Nelson, Stith, and Smedley 2003). Thus, even when blacks and Latinos have adequate health insurance, they still face barriers to high-quality care in the patient-provider relationship.

One way to overcome some of these racial barriers to health care equity is through advances in technology that allow people to utilize health care in new ways. Yet, little research has focused on whether the racial gap that exists for health care utilization also exists for accessing health information online and through mobile technologies. Recent research suggests that the racial technology gap may be less prominent once mobile technologies are examined (Ray, Gilbert, and Sewell 2016). Missing, however, is whether mobile technologies can help provide access to health information to reduce health disparities.

In this article, we use data from the Health Information National Trends Survey (HINTS) to examine racial differences in obtaining health information online via mobile devices. We first provide an overview of research on the racial gap in health care access and utilization. Second, we discuss why mobile technologies may be useful for bridging the racial gap in health care access. Third, we describe our data and methods. Then, we present our findings and conclude by discussing the policy implications our findings

---

1. See www.census.gov/content/dam/Census/library/publications/2015/demo/p60-253.pdf.

have for federally funded programs such as Medicaid, the Obama Phone Program,[2] and the Healthy Food Financing Initiative Bill.

Background

The Racial Digital Divide: Issues of Access

"Segregation concentrates economic disadvantage with racial disadvantage" (Ray, Gilbert, and Sewell 2016). Roughly 8 million Americans live in extreme poverty neighborhoods, with 40 percent of the local residents living below the poverty line. Due to housing segregation and discrimination, blacks and Latinos are more likely to live in segregated, poor neighborhoods (Charles 2003). Poor neighborhoods are often isolated from technological infrastructure that becomes useful for taking advantage of advances in health care. Mobile technologies allow for the use of health devices that require wireless technology (Wiehe et al. 2008). For example, pacemakers have wireless capabilities that alert physicians when a patient's heart goes into atrial fibrillation. People who live in a poor neighborhood without access to wireless Internet in their homes cannot take advantage of this technological advancement to monitor their arrhythmias and have a higher likelihood of stroke and heart disease (Go et al. 2001).

Thus, in many ways, racial segregation operates as a structural barrier to health information. Structural barriers constrain the formation of interpersonal relationships with other residents and local and national organizations that connect local residents with trusted health care providers. Consequently, the diffusion of health information into poor and minority communities that can increase health care utilization by taking advantage of cutting-edge policy prescriptions is inhibited (Szreter and Woolcock 2004). This is important considering research that shows that blacks and Latinos are more likely to seek neighborhood resources than individuals in more affluent neighborhoods (Barnes 2003, 2004). This line of research suggests that access is key rather than individual motivation.

Mobile Technologies to Circumvent Issues of Health Information Access

Mobile technologies are different from e-health technologies and may lend themselves to different groups across race and social class in nuanced ways that need to be assessed. Recent research shows that blacks and Latinos may be less likely to have a landline but more likely to have a mobile

2. See www.obamaphone.com/obamaphone-providers.

phone (Ray, Gilbert, and Sewell 2016). They also may be less likely to have home-based Internet but more likely to use the Internet on their mobile phones than whites. How and/or for what purposes people use mobile phone technologies are important questions that have yet to be addressed by extant research. Although many individuals may use mobile technologies for work and leisure, those who are cut off from broadband services may use these technologies for accessing government services, identifying places to deal with food insecurity, and searching the Internet for health information to circumvent the lack of access to health care services and information from health care professionals.

We propose that mobile technologies can serve as central nodes in a network to connect poor, minority, or rural individuals with information that can improve their health. For example, there is an abundance of research on mobile technology applications used to increase physical activity and reduce obesity (Cavallo et al. 2012; Keller et al. 2014; Tate, Jackvony, and Wing 2003, 2004). We believe giving individuals similar access to health information via mobile technologies is vital considering that over 40 percent of US households do not have landline phones (Blumberg and Luke 2014) and instead only have a mobile phone. However, having a mobile phone does not mean that a person has access to the Internet with that mobile phone. A sizable percentage of the US population, who are also more likely to be poor and minority, do not have access to online resources in the same way as others.[3]

Bridging the Access and Health Information Divide

So, how do mobile technologies help reduce racial health disparities? First, mobile technologies allow health care providers to maintain regular contact with their patients. Similarly, mobile technologies provide researchers a low-cost opportunity to keep participants informed and engaged about research studies (Ray, Gilbert, and Sewell 2016). Second, mobile technologies allow for more real-time health information to be gathered and used. For example, patients with diabetes can take their blood sugar and enter it into a mobile technology application to receive how much insulin to administer.[4] This is important considering that the US Pharmacopeia Medication Errors Reporting Program finds that roughly "50 percent of all medication errors involve insulin."[5] Half of these errors occur among individuals who are 60 years of age or older. This program reports that

3. See www.pewInternet.org/2015/04/01/us-smartphone-use-in-2015/.
4. This information was obtained from Vanderbilt University radiologist Dr. Laveil Allen.
5. See www.diabetesincontrol.com/a-review-of-insulin-errors/.

these errors add nearly $2,000 to a patient's total health care costs. As of 2014, over 29 million Americans had diabetes.[6] Without the use of these technologies, individuals on insulin continue to run the risk of giving themselves the wrong amounts of insulin. These errors can have grave implications for the patient by increasing morbidity and mortality, but also for state and federal budgets if the patient is on Medicaid or Medicare. This example illuminates how mobile technologies can increase communication between patients and health care providers, reduce costs, and improve overall health.

Third, mobile technologies may allow for patients with limited mobility and trouble accomplishing activities of daily living to interact with their health care providers without having to leave their homes (Vandelanotte et al. 2007). This type of technology is already being used for new mothers who have C-sections and may be limited in their ability to travel in the first month after birth. These technologies also decrease health care costs by reducing the number of days that patients may stay in the hospital. Furthermore, this type of mobile technology is being used by residents in Hawaii who may live on a different island from their health care provider. These types of technological advancements would be very useful for poor residents who have access issues due to limited public transportation routes or distance from health care providers.

With evidence documenting that blacks and Latinos are more likely to use mobile phone technology, coupled with individuals in economically disadvantaged neighborhoods aiming to access more social capital resources (Barnes 2003), there is reason to believe that blacks and Latinos may also use mobile technologies to access health information. We examine whether the digital divide exists for mobile technologies and whether such technologies lead individuals across racial and class divides to access health information in similar ways. While we do understand that accessing health information online is different from interacting with health care providers via mobile technologies, this examination is still fruitful as it may hold insights into ways to further circumvent racial disparities in health care access.

Methods

Data

We analyzed data from the Health Information National Trends Survey (HINTS) 4, Cycle 3. A cross-sectional, mail-administered survey, HINTS

---

6. See www.cdc.gov/diabetes/pubs/statsreport14/national-diabetes-report-web.pdf.

is designed to collect nationally representative data about the US population's health communication practices. Data were collected between September and December of 2013 with a response rate of 35.2 percent. A total of 3,165 respondents completed the portion of the survey that included the measures of interest. The sample was further restricted to include only respondents ages 18 to 59 who provided data on key independent variables (racial group membership, insurance type, mobile device access) and sociodemographic attributes. The age and race/ethnicity restrictions of the data account for the largest reductions in the sample size (roughly 42 percent). Although people over the age of 60 are more likely to face chronic diseases than the age group in our study, we assert that our study has the potential to help policy makers get ahead of ways to increase utilization as people age. Given that the study focused on multiple outcomes, the sample size varied slightly based on the outcome of interest. A total of 1,036 respondents provided valid data on all measures of interest.

Measures

Dependent Variables. The primary dependent variables were ascertained from a series of questions concerning attitudes and behaviors toward the sources of health information. Trust in sources of health information was ascertained from the following question: "In general, how much would you trust information about health or medical topics from [source]?" Twelve sources of health information were evaluated: (1) doctor; (2) family or friends; (3) online newspapers; (4) print newspapers; (5) special health or medical magazines or newsletters; (6) radio; (7) internet; (8) local TV; (9) national or cable TV news programs; (10) government health agencies; (11) charitable organizations; and (12) religious organizations and leaders. The four response options included: not at all; a little; somewhat; very. Higher responses indicate more trust. In some analysis, the values were recoded so that higher values indicated trust in the source of health information.

Among people who reported having "ever looked for information about health or medical topics from any source," recent source of health information was ascertained from the following question: "The most recent time you looked for information about health or medical topics, where did you go first?" The response options were: (1) doctor or health care provider; (2) internet; (3) other (books; brochures, pamphlets, etc.; cancer organization; family; friend/co-worker; library; magazines; newspapers; telephone information number; complementary, alternative, or unconventional practitioner; other). A fourth response option was allowed for people who had not recently sought health information. A four-category outcome was created, as follows: (1) doctor or health care provider; (2) internet; (3) other (list); (4) did not seek health information recently.

Go-to source of health information was ascertained from the following question: "Imagine that you had a strong need to get information about health or medical topics. Where would you go first?" The response options were: (1) doctor or health care provider; (2) internet; (3) other (books; brochures, pamphlets, etc.; cancer organization; family; friend/co-worker; library; magazines; newspapers; telephone information number; complementary, alternative, or unconventional practitioner; other). A binary indicator of reliance on the Internet was also created by coding internet as 1 and all other non-missing responses as 0.

Table 1 provides a description of the variables used in the primary analysis based on the sample of individuals with non-missing data on all outcomes and covariates of interest. For convenience sake, trusting attitudes were dichotomized such that 1 = very trusting; 0 = not at all, a little, or somewhat trusting. All other measures are reported in accordance with how they are used in the analysis.

Independent Variables. The analysis focused on explaining variation in the outcomes of interest due to three factors: (1) mobile device access; (2) insurance type; and (3) racial group membership. For mobile devices, we created a three-category ordinal measure to proxy mobile device access, where: (1) I do not have any of the above ("no mobile device"); (2) tablet computer only, smartphone only, or cell phone only ("1 mobile device"); and (3) multiple devices selected ("2+ mobile devices"). Mobile devices exclude desktop computers and laptops, but do include: tablets like an iPad, Samsung Galaxy, Motorola Xoom, or Kindle Fire; smartphones such as an iPhone, Android, Blackberry, or Windows Phone; and cell phones. This measure captured the relative extent to which a respondent was connected to the Internet via mobile devices. Higher values indicate more ways in which an individual can access the Internet.

For insurance type, we created a three-category nominal variable, where (1) no health care insurance; (2) Medicare, Medicaid, or any other; or (3) employer-provided or insurance purchased directly from an insurance company. All other responses were coded to missing. Of those that were missing, forty-nine respondents did not provide data on health care coverage, and seventy-six respondents reported some other form of health care insurance coverage than ascertained in this study (e.g., VA). Racial group membership was a self-reported measure and includes those who identify

Table 1   Weighted Means of Outcomes of Interest, Independent Variables, and Sociodemographic Attributes, Ages 18–59, HINTS 4 – Cycle 3, $N=1,036$

	Black	Latino	White
Outcomes of Interest			
Sources trusted for health information			
Doctor	0.71	0.70	0.70
Family	0.10	0.03	0.06
Online news sources	0.02[b]	0.09[a]	0.03
Print news sources	0.01	0.06[a]	0.02
Health news sources	0.28	0.27	0.23
Radio	0.02[a]	0.04[a]	0.01
Internet	0.15	0.12	0.11
Local TV	0.05	0.08[a]	0.02
National TV	0.05	0.10[a]	0.04
Government	0.35	0.32	0.28
Charities	0.12	0.12[a]	0.05
Religious organization	0.06[a]	0.08[a]	0.03
Sought health information recently from . . .			
The internet	0.49[a]	0.50[a]	0.67
Doctor or health care provider	0.13	0.06	0.07
Other sources	0.11	0.14[a]	0.08
Not sought information recently	0.26	0.31	0.18
In need of health information, would go to . . .			
The internet	0.37[a]	0.45	0.52
Doctor or health care provider	0.56[a]	0.49	0.41
Other source	0.07	0.06	0.07
Independent Variables			
Mobile device access			
No mobile devices	0.07	0.13[a]	0.03
1 Mobile device	0.47	0.33	0.43
2+ Mobile devices	0.46	0.54	0.54
Insurance type			
Federally insured	0.23[a]	0.14	0.10
Only privately insured	0.54[a]	0.50[a]	0.72
Uninsured	0.23	0.36[a]	0.19
Sociodemographic Controls			
Male (0 = Female)	0.44	0.55	0.49
Age	39.14	37.55	39.45
Geographical region			
Midwest	0.23	0.06[a]	0.25
South	0.53[a]	0.40	0.33
West	0.06[a,b]	0.32	0.25
Northeast (ref.)	0.18	0.21	0.17

Table 1   (*continued*)

	Black	Latino	White
Marital status			
Divorced/widowed/separated	0.13	0.08	0.12
Single	0.43[a,b]	0.23	0.26
Married/cohabitating (ref.)	0.44[a,b]	0.69	0.62
Total household size	3.21[b]	3.67[a]	3.09
Household income	70208	73647	78592
Highest education level			
Less than high school (ref.)	0.11[a]	0.17[a]	0.02
High school diploma	0.27	0.25	0.22
Some college	0.18[a]	0.21[a]	0.47
College degree	0.22	0.25	0.19
Graduate school	0.23[a]	0.13	0.10
Occupational status			
Employed (ref.)	0.72	0.66[a]	0.78
Unemployed	0.15[a]	0.12[a]	0.04
Not in labor market or retired	0.12	0.23	0.18
Felt sad . . .			
All of the time	0.01	0.00	0.01
Most of the time	0.02	0.04	0.04
Some of the time	0.30	0.24	0.21
A little of the time	0.42[a]	0.47	0.53
None of the time	0.25	0.25	0.21
Ever diagnosed with cancer	0.04	0.03	0.04
Self-rated health			
Poor	0.03[a]	0.02	0.01
Fair	0.21[a]	0.15	0.08
Good	0.28	0.40	0.34
Very good	0.37	0.29[a]	0.45
Excellent	0.12	0.14	0.12
N	172	201	663

[a]$p < .05$, statistically different from whites (two-tailed test).
[b]$p < .05$, statistically different from Latinos (two-tailed test).

as either white, black or African American, or Hispanic/Latino. Due to small sample sizes for other groups, they were excluded from the analysis.

Control Variables. Control variables included sociodemographic attributes and health. Sociodemographic attributes included gender, age, marital status, household size, household income (mid-repoint recode of nine-category ordinal variable with the following categories: $0 to $9,999;

$10,000 to $14,999; $15,000 to $19,999; $20,000 to $34,999; $35,000 to $49,999; $50,000 to $74,999; $75,000 to $99,999; $100,000 to $199,999; $200,000 or more), highest educational level in household, and occupational status. Health indicators included a five-category ordinal measure of feeling sad in the most recent month, lifetime cancer diagnosis, and self-rated health.

Analytic Strategy

We noted missing data for both the dependent and independent variables for the 18–59 population. Percentages with missing data for the dependent variables were low, ranging from 0.7 percent (trust in doctors) to 7.4 percent (recent source of health information). Percentages of respondents having missing data on independent variables ranged from 0.0 percent (geographical region, marital status) to 3.5 percent (occupational status). We assumed the data were missing at random, and deleted all cases from the list with missing data on independent variables allowing for variation in sample sizes based on the dependent variable of choice.

All analyses were adjusted for the complex survey design of HINTS. Survey estimation (svy:) commands in Stata 14 were used to include probability weights (person_finwt0), clustering by Designated Market Areas (dma), and three different sampling strata (stratum). Trust in sources of health information outcomes were measured using ordered logistic regression with an allowance for five response categories. For behaviors and attitudes toward the Internet as a source of health information, multinomial logistic regression was used with health care providers as the reference category. Wald tests for combining alternatives (Long and Freese 2014) were conducted to determine if there were differences in behaviors and attitudes toward sources of health information among the different types. These tests suggested that the Internet response option could not be combined with other nonmedical response options or with the Never category (for recent source of health information). The tests also revealed that health care providers could not be combined with other outcome responses. So, we analyzed three categories: Internet, health care providers, and other nonmedical sources.

In the analysis that follows, we provide four types of estimates. First, we include estimates of racial disparities in trusting twelve different sources of health information, holding constant sociodemographic attributes and health-related indicators. Second, we provide estimates of racial disparities in utilization behaviors and willingness attitudes toward the specified sources of health information, holding constant sociodemographic attributes and health-related indicators. Third, we provide estimates of racial disparities in attitudes toward the Internet as a go-to source of health information, while adjusting for the main and moderating effect of insurance type and for the main and moderating effect of mobile device access. Fourth, we provide estimates of racial disparities in attitudes toward the Internet as a go-to source of health information, while adjusting for the ways that insurance type moderates the main effect of mobile device access. For each type of evaluation with second-order interactions, we produced adjusted models that control for sociodemographic attributes, health-related indicators, and trust in the Internet as a source of health information (see figs. 1, 2, and 3).

Limitations

The data in our study obviously have limitations that impact our analysis. First, the survey had a low response rate. Though this response rate is similar to—and, in some regards, better than—other studies that sample using traditional phone methods, we do not have information for the potential respondents who opted out of the study either due to non-response or refusal. Therefore, there may be response bias present in the sample, though research is mixed on whether non-respondents differ from respondents in nationally representative and/or random samples (Abraham, Helms, and Presser 2009; Tourangeau, Groves, and Redline 2010). Second, we were unable to ascertain the specific types of websites and news sources that respondents obtained from the Internet. Third, it is possible that people who use their mobile devices to do Internet searches for health information may have unmeasured characteristics that also are associated with getting mobile devices in the first place, leading to endogeneity issues (e.g., doing Internet searches may make them care more about accessing health information than people who do not do those things). Fourth, although we purport that accessing health information online may translate to telehealth opportunities, assessing this potential payoff is beyond the scope of this study. We also do not want to imply that telehealth can be used as a substitute for direct interaction with health care providers. Rather, we view telehealth as another tool for health care providers to use, and the potential payoff from these opportunities may benefit individuals living in impoverished communities. Future research should aim to explore these possibilities given policy changes that aim to enhance wireless capabilities.

Table 2 Ordinal Logistic Regression for Trusting Sources of Health Information on Racial Group Membership, HINTS 4 – Cycle 3 (Whites Reference Group)

	Black	Latino	N
Doctor	1.09	0.96	1,194
	(0.26)	(−0.15)	
Family	0.89	0.49***	1,192
	(−0.38)	(−3.43)	
Online news	1.61*	1.66*	1,189
	(2.36)	(2.15)	
Print news	1.44+	1.06	1,181
	(1.76)	(0.30)	
Health news	1.35	1.08	1,194
	(1.06)	(0.30)	
Radio	1.67*	1.30	1,192
	(2.14)	(1.16)	
Internet	1.22	1.12	1,198
	(0.66)	(0.50)	
Local TV	1.87**	2.34***	1,185
	(2.69)	(3.53)	
National TV	1.99***	2.21**	1,191
	(3.38)	(3.31)	
Government	1.48+	1.54*	1,186
	(1.67)	(2.05)	
Charities	1.69+	1.48	1,187
	(1.96)	(1.44)	
Religious organizations	2.81***	1.34	1,190
	(4.73)	(1.30)	

Note: Exponentiated betas shown. Z-statistic in parentheses (two-tailed test). Models include controls for sociodemographic attributes, including male gender, age, geographical region, marital status, household size, household income, household education, occupational status, sadness in past month, cancer diagnosis, and self-rated health.

$+p < 0.10$, $*p < 0.05$, $**p < 0.01$, $***p < 0.001$ (two-tailed test)

Results

Racial Disparities in Trusting Sources of Health Information

Table 2 shows racial disparities in trusting twelve different sources of health information. The estimates adjust for racial differences in socio-demographic attributes that may also be correlates of trust. The analysis reveals heterogeneity in the nature and degree of black-white and Latino-white disparities in trust in sources of health information.

Blacks are more likely to trust health information from online news sources, radio, local TV, national TV, and religious organizations than whites, while Latinos are more likely to trust online news, local TV, national TV, and the government than whites. Latinos are less likely than whites to trust health information from family members; yet, no black-white differences exist in trusting this source of health information. In addition to there being no racial differences in trusting doctors for health information, there are also no racial differences in trusting print news, health news, the Internet, and charities. There are also no statistically significant black-white differences in trusting government, and no Latino-white differences in trusting religious organizations.

Racial Disparities in Use of and Reliance on the Internet for Health Information

Table 3 shows variation in recent use of the Internet and reliance on the Internet in times of strong need by racial group membership, insurance type, and mobile device access status—the key covariates of interest in this study. The results reveal that distrust in the Internet is associated with lack of use and reliance on the Internet as a source of health information. The estimates indicate that people who think the Internet is not a trust-worthy source of health information are less likely to actually have used the Internet in the most recent search for health information compared to using a doctor. They are also less likely to use the Internet as a go-to source for health information in times of strong need for information about health.

Holding constant distrust in the Internet, there are no racial differences in recent use of the Internet, but blacks are less likely than their white counterparts to rely on the Internet and other nonmedical sources. That is, blacks are more likely to report preferring to go to a doctor or health care provider during times of strong need. There are no Latino-white differences in either use of or reliance on the Internet.

There are, however, gaps in Internet use and reliance based on insurance type. Individuals who are insured by Medicare or Medicaid (i.e., federally insured) are less likely than the uninsured to use the Internet when looking for health information recently. In fact, insured persons (both federally and privately insured) are less likely than the uninsured to indicate the Internet as a go-to source of health information in times of strong need. There are no main associations with mobile device status, holding constant these key covariates of attitudes toward the Internet.

Table 3 Multinomial Logistic Regressions for Use of and Reliance on Internet for Health Information on Racial Group Membership, HINTS 4 – Cycle 3

	The Most Recent Time You Looked for Health Information, Where Did You Go First? (Reference: Provider)			Imagine You Had a Strong Need to Get Health Information, Where Would You Go First? (Reference: Provider)	
	Internet	Other	Never	Internet	Other
Black	0.37+	0.88	0.76	0.43**	0.32*
	(−1.83)	(−0.21)	(−0.53)	(−2.82)	(−2.12)
Latino	1.11	3.30+	1.69	0.70	0.45+
	(0.20)	(1.92)	(0.90)	(−1.24)	(−1.71)
Any federal	0.08*	0.26	0.14+	0.26***	0.84
	(−2.31)	(−1.25)	(−1.82)	(−3.41)	(−0.33)
Private only	0.19	0.40	0.18	0.27***	0.60
	(−1.62)	(−0.85)	(−1.62)	(−3.92)	(−1.03)
1 device	5.95+	1.61	1.24	2.17	0.90
	(1.92)	(0.55)	(0.26)	(1.29)	(−0.21)
2+ devices	4.66+	0.44	0.65	2.63	0.72
	(1.67)	(−0.85)	(−0.53)	(1.61)	(−0.55)
Distrust in Internet	0.24***	0.61+	0.70	0.32***	0.60*
	(−6.41)	(−1.77)	(−1.38)	(−6.80)	(−2.00)
N		1,086		1,198	

Note: Exponentiated betas shown. Z-statistic in parentheses (two-tailed test). Models include controls for sociodemographic attributes not shown, including male gender, age, geographical region, marital status, household size, household income, household education, occupational status, sadness in past month, cancer diagnosis, and self-rated health.
+$p < 0.10$, *$p < 0.05$, **$p < 0.01$, ***$p < 0.001$ (two-tailed test)

Differential Reliance on the Internet by Insurance Type across Racial Groups

Uninsured individuals of all races are more likely to rely on the Internet as their go-to source for health information. However, the gap between the uninsured and the privately insured is smaller for blacks and Latinos than among whites. Compared to whites, the uninsured/privately insured gap is 5.92 times smaller among blacks ($z = 2.74$) and 3.65 times smaller among Latinos ($z = 2.54$) (table 4, column 1). These race differentials in the relative association of insurance type with reliance on the Internet hold when adjusting for sociodemographic attributes (fig. 1; table 4, column 2).

Table 4 Logistic Regression for Reliance on Internet on Racial Group Membership, Insurance Type, and Mobile Device Access, HINTS 4 – Cycle 3

	Racial Group Membership X Insurance Type		Racial Group Membership X Mobile Device Access		Insurance Type X Mobile Device Access	
	Unadjusted	Adjusted	Unadjusted	Adjusted	Unadjusted	Adjusted
Black	0.16**	0.18*	0.02**	0.02***	0.63+	0.53*
	(−3.11)	(−2.59)	(−3.03)	(−3.65)	(−1.76)	(−2.26)
Latino	0.34*	0.40+	0.26	0.12+	0.84	0.82
	(−2.30)	(−1.92)	(−1.22)	(−1.90)	(−0.73)	(−0.72)
Any federal	0.33*	0.26**		0.24***	8.19+	10.88*
	(−2.25)	(−2.78)		(−3.57)	(1.80)	(2.09)
Private only	0.40**	0.20***		0.28***	0.79	0.60
	(−3.00)	(−4.37)		(−4.18)	(−0.21)	(−0.48)
1 Device		2.03	2.26	1.01	10.66**	9.13*
		(1.30)	(1.22)	(0.02)	(2.69)	(2.39)
2+ Devices		2.46+	3.11+	1.31	24.82***	10.60*
		(1.65)	(1.68)	(0.39)	(3.59)	(2.49)
Black X any federal	2.65	1.97				
	(1.20)	(0.79)				
Latino X any federal	0.78	0.59				
	(−0.31)	(−0.60)				
Black X private only	5.92**	4.15*				
	(2.74)	(2.08)				
Latino X private only	3.65*	3.10*				
	(2.54)	(1.99)				

(continued)

Table 4 Logistic Regression for Reliance on Internet on Racial Group Membership, Insurance Type, and Mobile Device Access, HINTS 4 – Cycle 3 (continued)

	Racial Group Membership X Insurance Type		Racial Group Membership X Mobile Device Access		Insurance Type X Mobile Device Access	
	Unadjusted	Adjusted	Unadjusted	Adjusted	Unadjusted	Adjusted
Black X 1 device			17.01*	17.77*		
			(2.19)	(2.58)		
Latino X 1 device			4.06	11.32*		
			(1.23)	(1.99)		
Black X 2+ devices			36.60**	39.45**		
			(2.70)	(3.29)		
Latino X 2+ devices			3.14	4.97		
			(1.05)	(1.46)		
Any federal X 1 device					0.04**	0.01***
					(−2.64)	(−3.40)
Private only X 1 device					0.79	0.47
					(−0.21)	(−0.67)
Any federal X 2+ devices					0.03**	0.02**
					(−2.86)	(−2.99)
Private only X 2+ devices					0.48	0.49
					(−0.66)	(−0.66)
N	1,198	1,198	1,198	1,198	1,198	1,198

Note: Exponentiated betas shown. Z-statistic in parentheses (two-tailed test). Adjusted models include controls for mobile device access, trust in the Internet, and sociodemographic attributes, including male gender, age, geographical region, marital status, household size, household income, household education, occupational status, sadness in past month, cancer diagnosis, and self-rated health.
$+p < 0.10$, $*p < 0.05$, $**p < 0.01$, $***p < 0.001$ (two-tailed test)

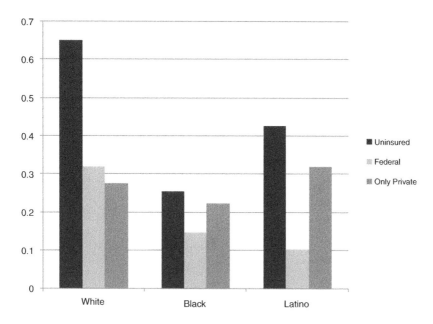

Figure 1   Predicted Likelihood of Internet as Go-To Source of Health Information When in Need by Race and Insurance Type, Adjusted Model

Differential Reliance on the Internet by Mobile Device Access across Racial Groups

Having a mobile device is associated with reliance on the Internet as a go-to source of health information for all racial groups. However, the relative extent to which the mobile device divide matters for Internet health information reliance varies by racial group. For instance, there is a smaller gap between people who have two or more mobile devices and people who have no mobile device among whites than among either blacks or Latinos (table 4, column 3). Blacks who do not have a mobile device face a serious dearth of reliance on the Internet. Virtually no blacks in these data who did not have a mobile device reported that they would turn to the Internet for health information in a time of need (fig. 2; table 4, column 4). The probability of Internet reliance of Latinos who are not connected is only slightly higher than the comparable probability for blacks. Even though connected blacks are less likely to rely on the Internet than connected whites, the large magnitude of the mobile device divide between blacks with no devices, compared to one or two devices, indicates that being connected

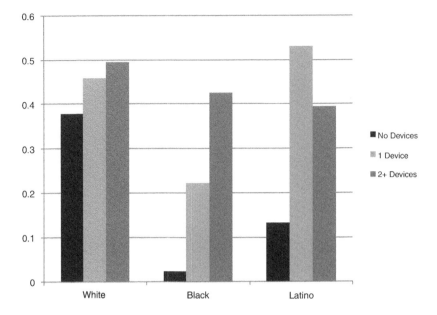

Figure 2 Predicted Likelihood of Internet as Go-To Source of Health Information by Race and Mobile Device Access, Adjusted Model

provides blacks with a vastly different orientation toward the Internet and its relationship with health information than is the case among whites.

Differential Reliance on the Internet by Mobile Device across Insurance Types

Having a mobile device is associated with reliance on the Internet as a go-to source of health information for all insurance types. However, the relative extent to which the mobile device divide matters for Internet health information reliance varies by insurance type. For instance, there is a larger gap between people who have two or more devices and people who have no mobile devices among the uninsured and the privately insured than among the federally insured (table 4, column 5). Holding constant socio-demographic attributes, federally insured persons who do not have a mobile device are more likely to rely on the Internet as a go-to source for health information than uninsured and privately insured persons who have one mobile device (fig. 3; table 4, column 6). These findings indicate that

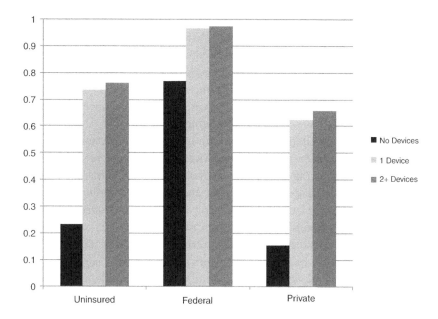

Figure 3   Predicted Likelihood of Internet as Go-To Source of Health Information by Insurance Type and Mobile Device Access, Adjusted Model

the mobile device divide is nearly nonexistent among federally insured persons, but is prominent among people who lack insurance and people who have private insurance. Mobile devices may serve similar functions for the uninsured and the privately insured.[7]

Health Policy Implications

Establishing health equity for all Americans regardless of race/ethnicity or social class background is not solely about economic resources. Rather, health equity is also about social resources and providing individuals with the ability to exert agency to maintain and improve their health outcomes. Providing access to health information allows people to obtain knowledge important to their well-being more expeditiously. Health information dissemination improves health literacy and may enhance compliance and

7. Supplemental analysis (available upon request) examined the probability of a three-way interaction between racial group membership, mobile device access, and insurance type; however, sample sizes for minorities were too small to conduct a reliable test of third-order interactions.

behavioral change. It also allows people to become more prepared for interactions with health care providers and feel greater autonomy over their lives. For people with chronic health conditions such as diabetes, heart failure, and kidney failure, mobile and wireless technologies allow them to maintain care in outpatient settings rather than in hospital settings. This change in setting helps to reduce health care costs for insurance companies and government-sponsored insurance programs.

Despite these benefits, poor and minority community members are less likely to have access to mobile and wireless technology, yet more likely to have chronic health conditions. Providing wireless infrastructures to improve telehealth capabilities in poor and minority communities could help to overcome the lack of health care providers and inadequate resources in such neighborhoods. With these infrastructures, mobile technologies may be used to document how travel patterns and neighborhood locations are associated with health-risk behaviors across the life course of youth and aging adults. Nonetheless, providing access to mobile and wireless technologies is not a substitute for dealing with the real challenges of building an infrastructure of health that provides equitable opportunities for health care. Moreover, access to health information via mobile technology is simply a complement to primary care services for the underserved. Strategies that provide ways to enhance patient agency, while also aiming to overhaul an inequitable health care system, should be pursued simultaneously.

One health policy program, in particular, may lend itself to leveraging mobile technology for poor Americans. The Obama Phone Program allows residents who meet a certain financial threshold to obtain a mobile phone to communicate with employers, job prospects, and family members and friends. These phones, however, only give a person the ability to call and text. What is needed is the ability to gain access to the Internet. As we show here, blacks and Latinos will definitely heed these opportunities to access the Internet in order to obtain vital health information. Incentives and subsidies can be offered to corporations that provide wireless infrastructure in poor neighborhoods. This is in line with Healthy People 2010 objectives that aimed to increase the number of people with home-based Internet.

Altogether, mobile technologies are vital for health care as we progress into the twenty-first century. Finding ways to enhance existing programs in order to provide access to mobile technologies will correspondingly improve health literacy and outcomes. Mobile technologies may also contribute to reducing racial health disparities among whites, Latinos, and blacks, as well as those individuals on Medicare and Medicaid.

Conclusion

This article examined racial differences in the propensity to access health information online. Blacks and Latinos, compared to whites, were more likely to trust online newspapers to get health information. Blacks also were more likely than whites to use the Internet to access health information when in the midst of a strong need event. However, minorities who are privately insured were more likely than their uninsured counterparts to rely on the Internet. These findings are important considering that federally insured persons who are connected to mobile devices had the highest probability of reliance on the Internet as a go-to source of health information. In sum, these findings lend credence that mobile technologies are important for achieving greater racial equity in health behavior and health outcomes.

▪ ▪ ▪

Rashawn Ray is associate professor of sociology and the Edward McK. Johnson Jr. endowed faculty fellow at the University of Maryland (UMD), College Park. Formerly, Ray was a Robert Wood Johnson Foundation Health Policy Research Scholar at the University of California, Berkeley/UCSF. Ray's research addresses the mechanisms that manufacture and maintain racial and social inequality. His work also speaks to ways that inequality may be attenuated through racial uplift activism and social policy. Selected as a member of "40 under 40 Prince George's County" (Maryland), Ray has published over forty books, articles, book chapters, and op-eds, and was awarded the 2016 UMD Research Communicator Award.
rjray@umd.edu

Abigail A. Sewell is assistant professor of sociology at Emory University. Her research focuses on the political economy of racial health disparities; the interrelatedness of the economy, public policy, and racial domination; and quantitative methods in studies of race and supra-individual racism. Her work has received support from the National Institutes of Health, the Ford Foundation, the National Science Foundation, and the Society for the Study of Social Problems. Her work has been published in *Social Science Medicine*, *Social Science Research*, and *Journal of Urban Health*. She teaches courses in race, racism, and quantitative approaches in studies of ethnoraciality.

Keon L. Gilbert is an associate professor at the Saint Louis University College for Public Health and Social Justice, Department of Behavioral Sciences and Health Education. His primary research interests are inspired by a quest to reduce health disparities through chronic disease prevention and promoting healthy behaviors by applying mixed methods in areas such as social capital, community capacity, organizational readiness, and community-based participatory research with populations such as African American males. His research is centered on the intersection of racial and gender identity, racial and gender socialization, and structural racism as important, yet unexplored, determinants of African American males' health across the life course.

Jennifer D. Roberts is assistant professor of kinesiology at the University of Maryland, College Park, School of Public Health, and is the director of the Public Health Outcomes and Effects of the Built Environment (PHOEBE) Laboratory. Her research focuses on the relationship between the built environment and physical activity in addition to its impact on obesity and other public health outcomes. More specifically, much of her research has explored the dynamic relationship between environmental, social, and cultural determinants of physical activity, using empirical evidence of this relationship to infer complex health outcome patterns among adults and children.

Acknowledgments

The authors acknowledge the JHPPL special issue editors and reviewers as well as participants of the 2016 Robert Wood Johnson Foundation Investigator Awards conference for helpful comments on this manuscript.

References

Abraham, Katherine G., Sara Helms, and Stanley Presser. 2009. "How Social Processes Distort Measurement: The Impact of Survey Nonresponse on Estimates of Volunteer Work in the United States." *American Journal of Sociology* 114: 1129–65.

Barnes, Sandra L. 2003. "Determinants of Individual Neighborhood Ties and Social Resources in Poor Urban Neighborhoods." *Sociological Spectrum* 23, no. 4: 463–97.

Barnes, Sandra L. 2004. "Too Poor to Get Sick? The Implications of Place, Race, and Costs on the Healthcare Experiences of Residents in Poor Urban Neighborhoods." *Chronic Care, Healthcare Systems and Services Integration: Research in the Sociology of Healthcare* 22: 47–64.

Blumberg, Stephen J., and Julian V. Luke. 2014. "Wireless Substitution: Early Release of Estimates from the National Health Interview Survey, January–June 2014."

US Department of Health and Human Services. Centers for Disease Control and Prevention. National Center for Health Statistics. 1–14.

Boardman, Jason D., Jarron M. Saint Onge, Richard G. Rogers, and Justin T. Denney. 2005. "Race Differentials in Obesity: The Impact of Place." *Journal of Health and Social Behavior* 46: 229–43.

Cavallo, David N., Deborah F. Tate, Amy V. Ries, Jane D. Brown, Robert F. Devellis, and Alice S. Ammerman. 2012. "A Social Media-Based Physical Activity Intervention: A Randomized Controlled Trial." *American Journal of Preventive Medicine* 43, no 5: 527–32.

Charles, Camille Z. 2003. "The Dynamics of Racial Residential Segregation." *Annual Review of Sociology* 29: 167–207.

Diez-Roux, A. V. 2001. "Investigating Neighborhood and Area Effects on Health." *American Journal of Public Health* 91: 1783–89.

Diez-Roux, Ana V. 2011. "Complex Systems Thinking and Current Impasses in Health Disparities Research." *American Journal of Public Health* 101: 1627–34.

Gilbert, Keon L., Rashawn Ray, and Marvin Langston. 2014. "Social Dis(ease) of African American Males and Health." In *Urban Ills: Twenty-First-Century Complexities of Urban Living in Global Contexts*, vol. 2., edited by Carol Camp Yeakey, Vetta Sanders Thompson, and Anjanette Wells, 23-36. Lanham, MD: Lexington Books.

Gilbert, Keon, Rashawn Ray, Arjumand Siddiqi, Derek Griffith, Elizabeth Baker, Shivan Shetty, and Keith Elder. 2016. "Visible and Invisible Trends in African American Men's Health: Pitfalls and Promises." *Annual Review of Public Health* 37: 295–311.

Go, Alan S., Elaine M. Hylek, Kathleen A. Phillips, YuChiao Chang, Lori E. Henault, Joe V. Selby, and Daniel E. Singer. 2001. "Prevalence of Diagnosed Atrial Fibrillation in Adults—National Implications for Rhythm Management and Stroke Prevention: The AnTicoagulation and Risk Factors in Atrial Fibrillation (ATRIA) Study." *Journal of the American Medical Association* 285, no. 18: 2370–75.

Hajat, A., J. S. Kaufman, K. M. Rose, A. Siddiqi, and J. C. Thomas. 2010. "Do the Wealthy Have a Health Advantage? Cardiovascular Disease Risk Factors and Wealth." *Social Science and Medicine* 71: 1935–42.

Kawachi, Ichiro, and Lisa F. Berkman. 2003. *Neighborhoods and Health*. New York: Oxford University Press.

Keller, Brett, Alain Labrique, Kriti M. Jain, Andrew Pekosz, and Orin Levine. 2014. "Mind the Gap: Social Media Engagement by Public Health Researchers." *Journal of Medical Internet Research* 16, no. 1: e8.

Kwate, Naa Oyo A., Chun-Yip Yau, Ji-Mengh Loh, and Donya Williams. 2009. "Inequality in Obesigenic Environments: Fast Food Density in New York City." *Health and Place* 15: 364–73.

Long, J. Scott, and Jeremy Freese. 2014. *Regression Models for Categorical Dependent Variables Using Stata*. College Station, TX: Stata.

Massey, Douglas S., and Nancy Denton. 1993. *American Apartheid: Segregation and the Making of the Underclass*. Cambridge, MA: Harvard University Press.

Nelson, Alan R., Adrienne Y. Stith, and Brian D. Smedley, eds. 2002. *Unequal Treatment: Confronting Racial and Ethnic Disparities in Health Care.* Washington, DC: National Academies.

Ray, Rashawn, Keon L. Gilbert, and Abigail A. Sewell. 2016. "Mobile Technology as a Conduit for Reducing Obesity-Related Health Disparities." *Issues in Race and Society* 4, no. 1: 98–119.

Sewell, Abigail A. 2010. "A Different Menu: Racial Residential Segregation and the Persistence of Racial Inequality." In *Race and Ethnic Relations in the 21st Century: History, Theory, Institutions, and Policy*, edited by Rashawn Ray, 279–90. San Diego: Cognella Publishing.

Sewell, Abigail A. 2015. "Disaggregating Ethnoracial Disparities in Physician Trust." *Social Science Research* 54: 1–20.

Stainback, Kevin, and Donald Tomaskovic-Devey. 2012. *Documenting Desegregation: Racial and Gender Segregation in Private-Sector Employment Since the Civil Rights Act.* New York: Russell Sage Foundation.

Szreter, Simon, and Michael Woolcock. 2004. "Health by Association? Social Capital, Social Theory, and the Political Economy of Public Health." *International Journal of Epidemiology* 33, no. 4: 650–67.

Tate, Deborah F., Elizabeth H. Jackvony, and Rena R. Wing. 2004. "Effects of Internet Behavioral Counseling on Weight Loss in Adults at Risk for Type 2 Diabetes: A Randomized Trial." In *Year Book of Psychiatry and Applied Mental Health*, 96–97.

Tate, Deborah F., Elizabeth H. Jackvony, and Rena R. Wing. 2003. "Effects of Internet Behavioral Counseling on Weight Loss in Adults at Risk for Type 2 Diabetes." *Journal of the American Medical Association* 289, no. 14: 1833–36.

Tourangeau, Roger, Robert M. Groves, and Cleo D. Redline. 2010. "Sensitive Topics and Reluctant Respondents: Demonstrating a Link between Nonresponse Bias and Measurement Error." *Public Opinion Quarterly* 74: 413–32.

Vandelanotte, C., K. M. Spathonis, E. G. Eakin, and N. Owen. 2007. "Website-Delivered Physical Activity Interventions: A Review of the Literature." *American Journal of Preventive Medicine* 33, no. 1: 54–64.

Wiehe, Sarah E., Shawn C. Hoch, Gilbert C. Liu, Aaron E. Carroll, Jefery S. Wilson, and J. Dennis Fortenberry. 2008. "Adolescent Travel Patterns: Pilot Data Indicating Distance from Home Varies by Time of Day and Day of Week." *Journal of Adolescent Health* 42: 418–20.

Williams, David R., and Chiquita Collins. 1995. "U.S. Socioeconomic and Racial Differences in Health." *Annual Review of Sociology* 21: 349–86.

Cautious Citizenship: The Deterring Effect of Immigration Issue Salience on Health Care Use and Bureaucratic Interactions among Latino US Citizens

Franciso I. Pedraza
University of California, Riverside

Vanessa Cruz Nichols
University of Michigan

Alana M. W. LeBrón
University of California, Irvine

Abstract   Research shows that health care use among Latino immigrants is adversely affected by restrictive immigration policy. A core concern is that immigrants shy away from sharing personal information in response to policies that expand bureaucratic monitoring of citizenship status across service-providing organizations. This investigation addresses the concern that immigration politics also negatively influences health care utilization among Latino US citizens. One implication is that health insurance expansions may not reduce health care inequities among Latinos due to concern about exposure to immigration law enforcement authorities. Using data from the 2015 Latino National Health and Immigration Survey, we examine the extent to which the politics of immigration deters individuals from going to health care providers and service-providing institutions. Results indicate that Latino US citizens are less likely to make an appointment to see a health care provider when the issue of immigration is mentioned. Additionally, Latino US citizens who know someone who has been deported are more inclined to perceive that information shared with health care providers is not secure. We discuss how cautious citizenship, or risk-avoidance behaviors toward public institutions in order to avoid scrutiny of citizenship status, informs debates about reducing health care inequities.

Keywords   health, health care, policy, Latino, immigration

Introduction

A major challenge to reducing health care inequities is that the costs of health insurance and health care deter people from using health care

Pedraza's research was supported by the RWJF, Scholars in Health Policy Research Program. LeBrón's research was supported by University of Michigan National Center for Institutional Diversity.

Journal of Health Politics, Policy and Law, Vol. 42, No. 5, October 2017
DOI 10.1215/03616878-3940486   © 2017 by Duke University Press

services for which they are eligible. Policy designed to subsidize coverage and expand eligibility, such as the 2010 Patient Protection and Affordable Care Act (ACA), helps address this challenge. For example, by September 2015, two years since key coverage provisions of ACA were implemented, Karpman and Long (2015) report a 41 percent decrease in uninsured rates among non-elderly adults. However, they also report that inequities in uninsurance rates remain disproportionately high for Latinos (23 percent) relative to non-Latinos (7 percent), even in Medicaid expansion states (Karpman and Long 2015). Expansions and subsidies may fall short if implemented without adequately accounting for various social, economic, and political forces (Chin et al. 2007; Kilbourne et al. 2008; Minkler 2010). One line of research that attends to such complexity focuses on the relationship between immigration policy and health (Hacker et al. 2011; Rhodes et al. 2015).

Disparate paths of research addressing inequities in health care coverage (Castañeda and Melo 2014; DeRose, Escarce, and Lurie 2007; Joseph 2016), health care access and utilization (Beniflah et al. 2013; DeRose, Escarce, and Lurie 2007; Donelson 2015; Toomey et al. 2014), and health outcomes (Cavazos-Rehg, Zayas, and Spitznagel 2007; Miranda et al. 2011; Rhodes et al. 2015) conclude that immigration policy is health care policy. Studies pointing to this conclusion begin by noting that immigration politics structures health-related outcomes because nativity and citizenship criteria determine program eligibility (Gee and Ford 2011; Zimmermann and Fix 1998). A related claim is that policy exclusions lead immigrants to worry that using welfare programs, including public programs related to health, increases the risk that they or those they are close to will be detected or classified as an unauthorized immigrant, which may spoil efforts to adjust citizenship status, or result in deportation (Fix and Passel 1999; Park 2011). Scholars also contend that immigration and immigrant policies reinforce definitions of national belonging that conflate citizenship status and ethnicity, which then transfers stigma associated with unauthorized immigration to entire groups of people, regardless of their citizenship status (Chavez 2008; Fox 2016; Viruell-Fuentes, Miranda, and Abdulrahim 2012). These studies highlight the salience of immigration issues and suggest why some people might be cautious about sharing personal identifying information, even with health care providers.

These strands of research corroborate a narrative that immigrant advocates use in describing withdrawal from full engagement in public life among immigrants and their United States-born co-ethnics in response to anti-immigrant policies (Kalet 2009; National Council of La Raza 2014;

Vallejo 2010). However, evidence is sparse on the extent to which restrictive immigrant policy spills over to US citizens and their propensity to access health care services. The presumption has been that US citizens are not personally at risk in an environment of more exclusionary immigrant policies; therefore, their behavior surrounding health care services that they are eligible for should not be shaped by such policies. We also know very little about whether the concerns outlined above extend broadly to other service-providing bureaucracies, or deeply to the perceptions that citizens have about the integrity of health care professionals to guard their personal information. Reducing health care inequities may require the trust of patients at various steps in the provision of services, including the collection of basic demographic information that helps determine appropriate diagnosis, treatment, and access to needed social and health care resources.

To what extent does the salience of immigration issues deter US citizens from using health care services? Who expresses skepticism about sharing personal identifying information in health care settings? In the sections that follow, we answer these questions theoretically and empirically. We argue that one consequence of contemporary restrictive immigrant policies is that it psychologically conditions Latinos to navigate daily life around considerations of immigration policy for themselves, for those they are close to, and for members of their social networks. The growth in immigration enforcement bureaucracies charged with identifying and detaining people in the interior of the United States (Koulish 2010; Meissner et al. 2013), as well as efforts to police citizenship by officials outside of law enforcement (Sampaio 2015), facilitates a psychological aversion to immigration-related issues. We contend that the rise of a restrictive immigrant climate has taught even Latino US citizens to adopt strategies that minimize their risk of experiencing harassment associated with questions about their citizenship status.

Using a population-based survey experiment, we test the claim that immigration issue concerns structure one's willingness to seek medical attention. By priming concerns over "immigration issues," as opposed to "health insurance" policy concerns, we expect respondents to be less willing to engage with health care providers. When we refer to *priming*, we refer to raising the relevance and recency with which certain considerations become activated in one's working memory (Fiske and Taylor 1991; Taylor and Fiske 1978). As a broader analysis, we also compare the effects of priming "immigration issues" to other facets of quotidian life. Despite their US citizenship, we find Latinos exposed to the "immigration issues" cue shy away from engaging with doctors, police, and, to a lesser extent, educators. We also find that a personal connection to someone who has been deported is associated with the belief that personal information shared with health care providers is not secure. In the final section, we discuss implications of our study for addressing health care inequities.

Issue Publics, Policy Feedback, and the Immigration-to-Health-Care Link

Our core theoretical argument is that the issue of immigration guides the way that many Latinos think about and engage with health care resources. We contend that both Latino health care inequities and evaluation efforts aimed at addressing such inequities require an understanding of how immigration and health care policy overlap. Connections between restrictive immigration and health care policy in the US relay messages to Latinos that they are unwelcome in America, and this connection is sustained by a decades-long protracted salience of immigration politics for Latinos. In this section, we draw on the concept of issue publics, priming, and the framework of policy feedback to motivate hypotheses about the relationship between immigration and engagement with health care providers.

Immigration Issue Salience and Latinos

Rather than one public that is highly informed about politics in general, societies consist of smaller issue publics (Converse 1964; Key 1966). Demands on our time from other aspects of life are too onerous to afford attention to a wide range of politics (Rosenstone and Hansen 1993; Verba, Schlozman, and Brady 1995). But most people pay attention to one or two issues. Groups of individuals who pay close attention to an issue, such as health care or immigration, are attentive to these political issues because of their salience in day-to-day life. Compared to nonmembers, members of issue publics form strong attitudes about their issue and use that issue to orient their political behavior (Krosnick 1990). Moreover, information in the political environment that raises the salience and accessibility of particular considerations—what social psychologists call *priming* (Fiske and Taylor 1991; Taylor and Fiske 1978)—can stimulate information collection for those with intense interest in that issue (Hutchings 2003). Priming effects can also influence political judgments broadly. For example, Nicholson (2005) found that issues primed by statewide ballot initiatives frame the way people think about and choose candidates for federal offices, even when those issues are not featured in those contests or extend beyond the scope of responsibilities associated with those offices. These studies uncover the power of priming effects to transcend institutional boundaries, and suggest that members of issue publics may use their issue priorities to guide how they think about other issue areas.

For Latinos, the link between matters of immigration and matters of health care begins with the importance of immigration as an issue. Gallup's famed question that asks what is the "most important problem" facing the country indicates that from 1994 to 2016, a multiracial nationally representative sample of Americans infrequently mention "immigration" as the most challenging issue, with most years registering less than 10 percent.[1] Unlike the perennial worry over jobs and the economy, only at key moments such as the 2006 immigration rallies (19 percent), the 2007 congressional debates over national immigration reform (15 percent), and the 2014 surge in refugees from Central America seeking asylum in the United States (17 percent), did more than one in ten Americans point to immigration as most important. In contrast, at six different points from 2004 to 2012, the Pew Hispanic Center observed no fewer than 27 percent of US Latinos citing immigration as the top issue, with peaks of 37 percent in 2007 and 34 percent in 2012.[2] For about one in three Latinos, or three times as many compared to the general public, immigration is a chronically salient policy issue.

Latinos are a key constituency of the immigration issue public for a more basic reason. Fifty-two percent of Latino adults are foreign born, and 85 percent of all Latinos have at least one immigrant grandparent (Fraga et al. 2011). Migration into Latino communities in the United States has been sustained over a century, replenishing Latino ethnic identity and reviving anti-Latino nativist impulses (Gratton and Merchant 2015; Jiménez 2008). Unlike immigrants from various European countries, Latino incorporation traces through conquest in the 1800s, through migration preceding the Great Depression, to newcomers sponsored through the Bracero guest-worker program that operated from 1942 to 1964, and to present-day workers from Mexico and other Latin American countries responding to the demand for cheap labor in the United States since the 1970s (Gutiérrez 2004; Massey 2002).

The salience of immigration for Latino US citizens today also stems from their personal proximity to undocumented immigrants, who are the

---

1. www.gallup.com/opinion/polling-matters/196733/gallup-review-americans-immigration
-election.aspx.
2. www.pewresearch.org/fact-tank/2014/06/02/top-issue-for-hispanics-hint-its-not-immigration/.

focus of the most intense debates in immigration politics. A 2014 survey of Latinos (Lopez, Gonzalez-Barrera, and Krogstad 2014) by the Pew Hispanic Center found that 23 percent of US-born Latinos, and 31 percent of US-born children of at least one immigrant parent, reported personally knowing someone who had been detained for immigration-related reasons or deported in the past year. Responses collected one year later in the 2015 Latino National Health and Immigration Survey (LNHIS), a survey that the authors of this study helped to design and field, suggest a similar figure: 39 percent of Latino US citizens, inclusive of immigrants who are naturalized citizens, personally know someone who has been deported. A major implication of deep and widespread personal connections to the immigration experience is that Latino US citizens are chronically primed by immigration matters in everyday life, including matters related to health care.

The concepts of issue priming and issue publics help clarify the salience of immigration issues to Latinos and the potential connection to other issues. The key to understanding why immigration politics is an obstacle to reducing health care inequities is the historical overlap between immigration and welfare-state policies. The overlap between immigration and welfare policies reveals crucial lessons to Latinos about their place in America, both as suspect clients of the welfare-state, as well as default targets of immigration enforcement. Next, we draw on the concept of policy feedback to explain why immigration provokes a psychological aversion to engagement with health care-providing resources among Latinos.

Policy Feedback and Deterred Engagement with Health Care Providers

The policy feedback framework posits that policy creates new politics by influencing mass publics through "resource" and "interpretive" effects (Pierson 1993). Policy investments in senior citizens (Campbell 2002) and veterans (Mettler 2005), for example, redistribute resources such as money and time, which facilitate political participation. Policy also has interpretive effects that can reshape later rounds of policy processes by empowering some voices and discouraging others. Interpretive policy effects begin simply with policy that classifies people and codifies criteria, such as nativity and citizenship, that determines who receives benefits and who receives burdens (Schneider and Ingram 1993). Policy also imparts lessons through participation in public programs that signal who is a deserving member of the polity (Soss 2002). Programs such as the GI Bill (Mettler 2005), Social Security (Campbell 2007), and Head Start (Soss 2002), teach people that government is responsive, and empower participants to engage in civic life. By contrast, "stop-and-frisk" policies and "show-me-your-papers" laws that disproportionately target blacks and Latinos communicate to members in those groups that government is not responsive to their needs and they are second-class members of society. Studies show that such laws nudge Latinos and blacks to distrust and avoid government (Burch 2013; Rocha, Knoll, and Wrinkle 2015; Walker 2014; Weaver and Lerman 2010). Here, we are interested in the interpretative lessons Latinos might glean from immigration policies and policies related to the provision of health care.

The social construction of immigrants and Latinos as less deserving stems from nineteenth-century public charge laws used to regulate entry into the United States. The United States is a nation that welcomes immigrants, the reasoning goes, but the United States must secure its own welfare before aiding the less fortunate of other nations. Public charge laws also exclude persons alleged to have committed or convicted of a crime, a provision lawmakers connected to Mexican immigrants in the debates that produced the 1924 Johnson-Reed Act (Ngai 2004). Importantly, Johnson-Reed introduced the concept of *illegal alien* (Ngai 2004: 58), which "Europeans and Canadians tended to be disassociated from," but "became constitutive of a racialized Mexican identity and of Mexicans' exclusion from the national community and polity."[3] From the perspective of policy feedback, overlap between immigration and welfare-state policies reifies nativity and citizenship as markers that distinguish more from less "deserving" groups (Myers 2007). Policy feedback theory anticipates that products of past policy, such as the designation of *illegal immigrant* and public charge rules, can have long-lasting influence on future policy outcomes and how subsets of the population view government.

The policy roots of health care inequities that grow from policing citizenship and nativity remain with us today. For example, the ACA continues to invoke citizenship and nativity as boundaries of our social obligations (Joseph 2016). Specifically, the health care exchanges created through the ACA call for local bureaucrats and computer systems to flag the citizenship status of applicants. The ACA systems are extensions of exclusions

---

3. Consuls applied such laws in the 1900s to exclude Mexicans (Daniels 2005). As evidence that stereotypes of Latinos as lazy and criminal spread via bureaucratic practice, Fox (2012) cites public charge data from the US Bureau of Immigration showing that between 1906 and 1932, Mexicans were deported at a higher rate than any other *single* nationality group.

codified in the 1996 Personal Responsibility, Work Opportunity and Reconciliation Act (PRWORA), which reinforced citizenship and nativity-based privilege by barring immigrants with authorized US presence who arrived after the law passed from accessing public benefits for five years or until attaining proper status. Although numerous states countered the five-year residency ban by legislating immigrants back into the fold within their jurisdiction, the 1996 federal bar initially excluded authorized immigrants from Medicaid, the Supplemental Nutrition Assistance Program, and Supplemental Security Income. States have implemented similar exemptions to cover excluded populations under the ACA. Still, contemporaneous to PRWORA are policies such as the 1996 Illegal Immigration Reform and Immigration Responsibility Act (IIRIRA), and the Anti-Terrorism and Effective Death Penalty Act (ATEDPA), which expanded US immigration enforcement powers by removing key components of due process for noncitizens, increasing the set of deportable crimes, and allowing retroactive application of deportation proceedings for crimes previously adjudicated (Welch 2002). Like PRWORA, IIRIRA and ATEDPA widen the gap in rights between noncitizen and citizen, setting the stage for the federal immigration enforcement of the 1990s that Watson (2014) and Vargas (2015) identify as deterring eligible people from using various welfare programs, including Medicaid.

More explicit ties between law enforcement officials and public health bureaucrats stretch back over a century. According to Molina (2006), rather than pointing to the unsanitary living conditions of labor camps provided by railroad companies, public health workers advanced racist claims of Mexicans' aversion to bathing to explain the spread of typhus in Los Angeles in 1916. After blaming Mexican immigrant railroad workers for typhus outbreaks, public health workers enacted policy that required railroad companies to quarantine new workers from Mexico and report the names of all new hires to the Los Angeles Board of Health. As Molina (2006: 66) explains, "[q]uarantine guards, invested with the same legal power as deputy sheriffs, policed the quarantine observation facilities to prevent anyone from leaving," and "the expanding information exchange between public agencies and private companies placed Mexicans under an unprecedented level of surveillance." Through their authority to implement health policy, public health officials associated themselves with immigration authorities. Ironically, by redirecting public health politics into immigration policy debates, health officials sowed the seeds of aversion toward their services, and potentially generated future Latino health care inequities.

Working with immigration authorities, relief bureaucrats divulged client information that guided mass deportation operations during the Great Depression. According to Fox (2012), Depression-era social workers ensured that poor European migrants settled into a world of relief and *inclusion*, while blacks in the South and Latinos in the Southwest, by contrast, faced *exclusion* from relief. For Mexicans and United States-born Mexican Americans, stakes mounted when charity workers passed applicant information to immigration officials that led to *expulsion* from the United States. As a strategy to thin welfare rolls, some relief agents like "the head of the Arizona Board of Public Welfare had no objections to letting immigration officers have access to the personal histories of all aliens applying for relief," while others like "the county board's lawyer advised against it, 'on the ground that many deserving aliens would be afraid to ask for help'" (Fox 2012: 151). As policy implementers, relief bureaucrats were aware of the "interpretive" effects—that is, the impact on public clients—of their choice to coordinate (or not) with immigration authorities. As targets of overlapping welfare and immigration policies, Latinos are very likely to have understood the stakes of turning to relief programs in this context, and gleaned a lesson to avoid public program participation.

Nativity- and citizenship-based exclusions from public program benefits are not limited to the Depression-era past; nor is cooperation between local welfare bureaucrats and federal immigration authorities. In 1994, California voters enacted Proposition 187, an initiative restricting undocumented immigrants from using public schools and public hospitals. The measure mandated that public workers report to officials any person they *suspected* of being undocumented. By interpreting "a discrete act of violating immigration law" as "a criminal tendency in Mexicans" (Jacobson 2008: 47), supporters of Proposition 187 reinforced the conflation of ethnicity with citizenship status, and revived the Depression-era practice of using local welfare bureaucrats as extensions of federal immigration enforcement authorities.

The courts deemed California's Proposition 187 unconstitutional. But, proponents left a legacy of arguments to justify policy prescriptions for public program exclusion and expulsion from the country, as well as reasoning to condone racial profiling as the means to achieve such ends. For instance, policy logic that conflates citizenship status with Latino identity motivated a health insurance fraud detection program targeting Latina women of child-bearing age at airports (Park 2011: 2). The California Department of Health Services initiated this fraud detection program, but it was discontinued in the early 2000s, according to Park (2011: 2), after investigators found program implementers "legally liable for overstepping the scope of their authority by attempting to influence federal [Immigration and Naturalization Services] decisions on whether to admit or deport immigrants as well as sharing confidential medical information in the process." Similarly, Proposition 187 replica legislation such as Arizona's S. B. 1070 (2010), Alabama's H. B. 56 (2011), and Georgia's H. B. 87 (2011) invoke the term "illegal alien" as justification for service-providing bureaucrats to identify suspected undocumented immigrants, sustaining the specter of racial profiling. Historically, policing citizenship happens at airports, welfare offices, and on the streets when encountering police—all contexts where personal information must be divulged.

Sensitivity to racial profiling and policing citizenship is particularly acute for Latinos following post-9/11 public investments in operations that focus on deporting people from the interior. According to the US Department of Homeland Security, the number of deportations from 2000 to 2015 exceeded the total number of deportations in the twentieth century.[4] Record-level deportations are possible, in part, because programs such as Secure Communities expand the geographic reach of immigration enforcement across and within each US state by coordinating federal and local law enforcement resources (Cox and Miles 2013; Meissner et al. 2013; Pedroza 2013). As evidence that Latinos have internalized policy lessons from Secure Communities operations—as predicted by policy feedback theory—Rocha, Knoll, and Wrinkle (2015) find that deportations increase distrust in federal and local government among both immigrant and US-born Latinos. Fueling criticism of interior-oriented immigration enforcement programs is evidence of racial profiling by local police, who identify and detain both Latino US citizens and persons without criminal records (Kohli and Chavez 2013; PBS 2011). In addition to bringing immigration authorities closer to their day-to-day life, interior operations are salient to Latinos because immigrants from Latin American countries represent 96 percent of all deportations from the United States since 2010 (TRAC 2014). In fact, after Arizona lawmakers passed a law mandating that local police officers inquire about immigration status during routine traffic stops (S. B. 1070), a 2010 survey of Latino voters in Arizona found that 72 percent said they believe that police primarily target Latinos (Barreto and Segura 2010). Subsequently, a 2011 survey of Latinos found that a majority of Latinos believe their group absorbs the brunt

---

4. www.dhs.gov/immigration-statistics/yearbook.

of restrictive immigration policies (Manzano 2011). For Latinos, mass deportation is not an abstraction, it is a reality that fuels worry for relatives, friends, coworkers, and students across Latino communities.

The literature links mistrust of health care providers and health care systems to health care inequities. These inequities are shaped by histories of institutional and interpersonal racism from medical institutions toward racial minorities, as well as racialized power imbalances between predominantly white health care providers and racial minority patients (Sewell 2015; Smedley, Stith, and Nelson 2003). In addition to the racializing role of public health institutions described above, studies indicate medical abuse of Guatemalans who were intentionally infected with syphilis and other infectious conditions in the 1940s (Reverby 2011), and the forced sterilization of Californians in the early- to mid-twentieth century (Stern et al. 2017). These medical and public health abuses serve to widen the structural space between Latinos and health care systems, which shapes patient mistrust of providers and public health institutions. Indeed, Sewell (2015) reports that Latino adults are more likely than non-Latino white adults to express mistrust in their health care providers' medical decision making and interpersonal competence. Similarly, qualitative research suggests that some undocumented immigrant youth perceive that physicians prioritize health care finances over medical decision making, contributing to mistrust in providers (Raymond-Flesch et al. 2014). This evidence base suggests that racial inequities in the mistrust of health care providers may contribute to health care inequities.

The arc from historical to contemporary accounts shows that immigration and public health policy streams compound one another to "position [Latinos] as a stigmatized out-group in American social cognition" (Massey 2013: 267). Past policy patterns that connect welfare stigma and social program deterrence give historical context to the 22 percent of Latinos in 2007 who indicated that they were less likely to use government services because of increased public attention to immigration issues (Pew Hispanic Center 2007: 18). Importantly, this figure is the same for immigrant and US-born Latinos, and was collected prior to the major expansions in interior-oriented immigration enforcement operations noted above (Golash-Boza 2012; Koulish 2010; Meissner et al. 2013). From the perspective of persons who are likely to be profiled, or who personally know someone who is likely to be profiled or has been deported, the interpretive lessons from contemporary immigration and welfare policy are that local law enforcement is not worthy of their trust, nor are the people and organizations who keep personal information that might be turned over to law enforcement officials. As Zayas (2015: 81) notes, in response to restrictive immigration policy, Latino communities "devise new ways of coping and techniques to evade the new restrictions and harsher penalties for immigration violations." Yet, as a source of factors that deter people from using health care services, we know very little about the extent to which the politics of immigration spills over to influence US citizens.

Hypotheses

Our central claim is that the overlap between welfare policy and immigration policy conditions Latinos to avoid service-providing bureaucracies, including health care-related services. We believe that interorganization cooperation that directs contact with welfare state officials to immigration enforcement authorities creates uncertainty about the intentions of social service bureaucrats. One plausible consequence of policy that creates uncertainty about interacting with social welfare organizations motivates our first and second hypotheses:

H1 Priming "immigration issues" deters Latino US citizens from using health care services.

H2 More generally, priming "immigration issues" provokes Latino US citizens' aversion to public service-providing officials.

We also argue that past experiences or anticipated experiences with deportation undermines the credibility of social service organizations to keep the personal information of clients secure. The historical and contemporary policy confluences produced by immigration politics and welfare politics teach Latinos, even those who are US citizens, to exercise caution in revealing, or at least to be sensitive to inquiries about, one's citizenship status or that of those with whom they are close. In the language of policy feedback, a potential interpretive effect of policing citizenship is that any bureaucrat who asks for personal identifying information may not be viewed as worthy of trust. We expect Latino US citizen attitudes about the security of personal information in the hands of health care providers to be conditional on proximity to undocumented immigrants. We hypothesize the following:

H3 Latino US citizens with personal connections to undocumented immigrants are more skeptical about the security of personal information shared with health care providers.

In the next section, we introduce a set of original survey questions that help us take a closer look at how immigration politics spills over to health care for Latino US citizens. Specifically, we use an experimental approach to evaluate the causal link between immigration and use of health care services, as well as other service-providing organizations. We complement this analysis with a probe of why some people might be cautious about sharing personal identifying information.

Data and Methods

We take advantage of the 2015 LNHIS, a survey sponsored in part by the Robert Wood Johnson Foundation Center for Health Policy at the University of New Mexico, as well as collaborating scholars from the University of Michigan at the time of the study implementation. Latino Decisions, a firm specializing in developing and fielding surveys of Latinos, implemented the survey and worked in conjunction with contributing scholars from multiple universities to design the survey instrument. The survey is uniquely designed to assess many of the most pressing health and health care concerns of the Latino community, as well as a wide range of matters related to the issue of immigration. The ability to evaluate attitudes about health, health care, and immigration issues with the same sample makes this an ideal dataset for our investigation.

The LNHIS (Total $N = 1,493$) relies on a sample provided by a mix of cell phone and landline households along with Web surveys. This mixed-mode approach improves our ability to capture a wide segment of the Latino population in the sample by providing a mechanism to poll the growing segment of the Latino population that lacks a landline telephone as well as those who prefer to engage surveys online. This approach is sensitive to some of the major shifts in survey methodology driven by changes in the communication behavior of the population. More specifically, the increasing number of Americans who have decided to use a cell phone for telephone communication while doing away with their landline telephone motivates our expansion of sample beyond landline households. A total of 989 Latinos were interviewed over the phone and an additional 504 Latinos were sampled through the Internet to create a dataset of 1,493 respondents. The Web-based respondents were randomly drawn from Latino Decision's national panel of Latino adults. The Web mode allows respondents to complete the survey in either English or Spanish, and contained the exact same questions as the telephone mode. Respondents from the Web are from a double-opt-in national Internet panel, and then randomly selected to participate in the study, and weighted to be representative of the Latino population.

All phone calls were administered by Pacific Market Research in Renton, Washington. The survey has an overall margin of error of ±2.5 percent with an American Association of Public Opinion Research response rate of 18 percent for the telephone sample. Latino Decisions selected Puerto Rico and the forty-four states with the highest number of Latino residents for the sampling design, which collectively account for 91 percent of the overall US Latino adult population. Respondents across all modes of data collection could choose to be interviewed in either English or Spanish. All interviewers were fully bilingual. Among those interviewed by phone, a mix of cell phone only (35 percent) and landline households (65 percent) were included in the sample, and the full dataset including both phone and Web interviews were weighted to match the 2013 Current Population Survey universe estimate of Latino adults with respect to age, place of birth, gender, and state. We use these weights in the statistical regression analysis below. The survey was approximately twenty-eight minutes long and was fielded from January 29, 2015, to March 12, 2015.

Our analysis is divided into three parts (one for each hypothesis), all of which focus on the 1,001 out 1,493 respondents who are Latino US citizens, either naturalized or by birth. We evaluate the first and second hypotheses using a subset of 732 out of the 1,001 participants who are US citizens and were included in a population-based survey experiment that we describe below in greater detail. The outcome variables of interest are self-reported health care use and engagement with other public service-providing organizations. We use all 1,001 participants who are US citizens to examine the third hypothesis about attitudes regarding the nature of personal information in health care settings. Specifically, we explore the correlates of the belief that information that patients disclose to health care professionals is shared with others rather than kept private and secure.

Results

Population-Based Survey Experiment: The Effect of Cueing Immigration Issues

We begin our analysis with a priming effect experiment administered to a representative sample of Latinos. This powerful design combines internal validity that rules out plausible alternative explanations with external validity that assures the observed effects exist in the population of interest as a whole (Mutz 2011). In a priming experiment, the aim is to compare whether exposure to a particular stimulus, in this case a phrase, influences responses to a later query. By randomly assigning respondents to either "health insurance" or "immigration issues" cues, we can compare which cue promotes or deters use of health care services, independent of other factors. We asked the following question: "When you are thinking about making an appointment to see a doctor or a nurse, or going to a clinic for health care, with all of the public attention to [issue prime], are you more likely to use health care services, less likely to use health care services, or it has not made a difference?"

Importantly, our selection of cues is designed to be subtle in two respects. First, because the items that are asked at the beginning of the 2015 LNHIS focus primarily on questions of health and health insurance (i.e., the ACA), the "health insurance" cue should provide continuity in the priming of considerations that prior survey items had already activated. For this reason, we anticipate that exposure to the phrase "health insurance" will activate considerations in a respondent's mind related to whether they have health insurance coverage, the costs of coverage, and perhaps the last visit to a health care provider or any wellness issue they are currently experiencing. Second, the "immigration issues" cue makes no explicit mention of immigration raids, detention, deportation, family separation, or any other outcomes associated with restrictive immigration policy. Instead, "immigration issues" also leaves open the possibility that expansive, welcoming, or otherwise positive considerations associated with immigration policy will be activated, including those related to "sanctuary cities," Deferred Action for Childhood Arrivals (DACA), Deferred Action for Parents of Childhood Arrivals (DAPA), and the Development, Relief, and Education for Alien Minors (DREAM) Act. For this reason, we anticipate that priming "immigration issues" will activate whatever balance of considerations a respondent holds in their memory about the issue of immigration.

If our claim that immigration provokes aversive responses is misguided, then we should see no difference in the reported anticipated use of health care services. In fact, our design does not preclude the possibility of observing the opposite, that "immigration issues" cues a greater expectation of using health care services. However, if simply mentioning the phrase "immigration issues" nudges US citizens to shy away from health care providers, then we will have identified evidence consistent with the "interpretive effects" that policy feedback scholars would theorize should occur in this case.

The evidence presented in fig. 1 shows that 29 percent of the respondents who were randomly assigned to receive the "health insurance" cue say that

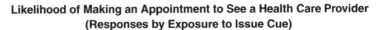

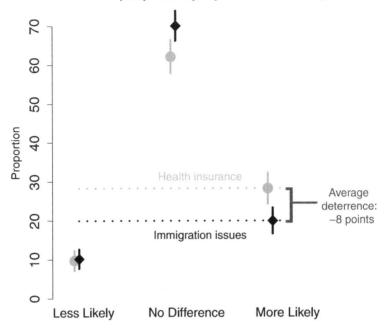

Figure 1 The Effect of Cueing "Health Insurance" versus "Immigration Issues" on the Propensity to Express Intention to See a Health Care Provider

they are "more likely" to make an appointment to see a health care provider. At 19 percent, the proportion expressing "more likely" is marginally fewer among respondents who were cued with "immigration issues" than for participants primed with the "health insurance" cue, about 8.4 percentage points lower (according to a chi-square test: $\chi^2 = 6.95$, $p = 0.03$; and according to a chi-square goodness of fit test: $\chi^2 = 12.99$, $p = 0.0015$). The difference in the effects of the cues is complicated by one point. About 70 percent of respondents cued with "immigration issues" say "no difference" in the likelihood of making appointments with health care providers compared to 62 percent who hear "health insurance," a difference of 7.9 points. Still, the 90 percent confidence intervals for each proportion estimate overlap considerably in the "less likely" responses and overlap a bit in the "no difference" responses. The lack of confidence interval overlap in the "more likely" responses indicates a statistically discernable effect. Although we observe stronger evidence for the aversion hypothesis, there does appear to be suggestive evidence of either a resilience or push-back response to the "immigration issues" cue among Latino US citizens.

Survey Experiment: Cautious Citizenship toward Public Service-Providing Institutions

The 2015 LNHIS data also allows us to extend our analysis of this experiment by comparing responses to questions that immediately followed the experiment. Here, we probe how far immigration politics is pushing Latinos to practice cautious citizenship, or exercise reticence to engage in the public sphere and with public service-providing institutions in order to avoid scrutiny of their citizenship status or that of their family members or social networks. Immediately following the priming experiment, we administered a battery of questions that is designed to measure the extent to which people are practicing cautious citizenship more broadly. The activities and behaviors include contact with police, educators, and, to facilitate comparison, health care providers, as well as a set of daily-life activities such as taking public transportation, picking up someone from the airport, driving a car, and renewing or applying for a driver's license. We find that one in six Latino US citizens avoid contact with service-providing bureaucracies, including police, educators, and health care providers. But does priming "immigration" induce aversion more broadly?

The magnitude of these effects is not trivial. On average, across the seven activities that we inquired about, 10 percent of Latino US citizens indicate avoidance when cued on "health insurance," as illustrated by the dashed gray line in fig. 2. For those exposed to the "immigration issues" cue, the average proportion expressing avoidance of daily-life activities in order to avoid questions about their citizenship status is 50 percent higher, or 5 percentage points higher, as marked by the dashed black line at 15 percent. Priming "immigration issues" is particularly consequential for engaging various service providers. People appear to be deterred from educators, health care providers, and police. The mere mention of *immigration issues* prompts about 20 percent of Latino US citizens to say that they avoid the police, compared to 12 percent who are primed with health insurance, approximately an eight-point difference. Corroborating what the main survey experiment indicated, we find that 10 percent of those exposed to the "health insurance" cue avoid health care providers, represented in fig. 2 with the x-axis label "clinic," versus 16 percent for those who were primed with "immigration issues."

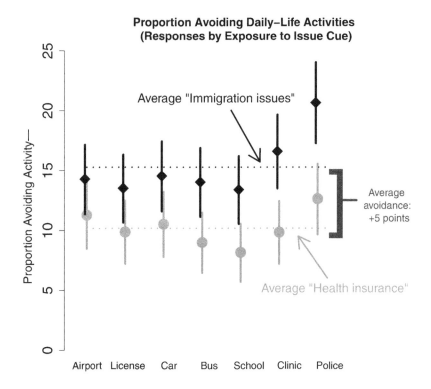

Figure 2 The Effect of Cueing "Health Insurance" versus "Immigration Issues" on the Propensity to Avoid Certain Daily-Life Activities in Order to Avoid Scrutiny about One's Citizenship Status

The strength of this part of our analysis is that we can make a direct comparison of priming effects to other areas of life. Table 1 shows that the "immigration issues" cue generates an aversive response across seven different areas of day-to-day life, and the differences in proportion for various public services are robust to several statistical tests. That avoidance effects are greatest for local law enforcement agencies is not surprising, because local police are increasingly implicated in the deployment of immigration enforcement operations that focus on identifying and detaining unauthorized immigrants in the interior of the country. However, when primed with the "immigration issues" cue, the extent of Latino US citizens' deterrence from health care providers (6 percent) is surprisingly similar to the avoidance reported with respect to police (8 percent), as shown in fig. 2.

Table 1 Tests of Difference in the Proportion of the Sample Who Report Avoiding Daily-Life Activities between Those Randomly Assigned to Receive the "Health Insurance" and "Immigration Issues" Condition

	χ^2	Kruskal-Wallis	Wilcox-Mann-Whitney	N
Airport	0.221	0.221	0.221	729
License	0.125	0.125	0.125	727
Car	0.101	0.101	0.101	725
Bus	0.033	0.033	0.033	727
School	0.023	0.023	0.023	721
Clinic	0.007	0.007	0.007	728
Police	0.004	0.004	0.004	720

Source: Data analyzed is a subset of the 732 US Latino citizens from the 2015 Latino National Health and Immigration Survey.
Note: Figures represent *p*-values.

Privacy of Health Information

Building on the answers to our first and second research questions, which suggest that after simply drawing their attention to the issue of immigration, Latino US citizens indicate that they will steer clear of health care providers and other public service bureaucrats, we turn next to assessing the depth of this disinclination in the context of health care. For our purpose here, we crafted an original survey question that simply asks: "Which of the following statements do you agree with most: Personal information I provide to my doctor and health care providers is secure and kept private; or, Personal information I provide to my doctor and health care providers is sometimes shared and not always secure?" In the statistical analysis below, we assign a value of 0 to those who believe personal information is private and secure, and assign a value of 1 to respondents who believe that information is shared and not always secure. We model the more skeptical view—that information is not always secure—using logistic regression.

Our main explanatory variables are nativity and proximity to persons vulnerable to immigration-related detentions or deportation. We use the following question to measure nativity: "Were you born in the United States, on the island of Puerto Rico, or in another country?" Although all of the respondents in our analysis are US citizens, this indicator, which we coded (0 = US born, 1 = foreign born), allows us to separate the foreign born who are likely to be more directly sensitive to immigration enforcement.

We include persons born on the island of Puerto Rico as US born, but conducted a robustness check and find no differences when categorizing Latinos born in Puerto Rico as born outside of the continental United States, in all models. Expulsion is one of the most coercive responses from the state, and we expect that experience with deportation, even if it is experienced indirectly through social connections, casts doubt on the assurances that any organization may claim about keeping personal information secure. To explore the "interpretive effects" of the historical overlap between immigration policies and health care bureaucracy practices, we include an indicator of whether someone personally knows an undocumented immigrant (coded 1 if yes, 0 otherwise). With these data we can also probe further with an indicator that distinguishes those who personally know someone who has been deported (coded 1 if yes, 0 otherwise).

Our question on the security of personal information was asked prior to the experiment that we reported above, so we are not concerned about the effect of priming "immigration issues" versus "health insurance." However, we do want control of factors that are likely to correlate with skepticism of personal information security. For example, given that the majority of people who are deported from the United States are from Mexico—according to TRAC (Transactional Records Access Clearinghouse) (2014) that figure is 69 percent in 2012 and 65 percent in 2013—we include an indicator for Mexican national origin, which we anticipate will be positively associated with a skeptical view. Because there is a stereotype that Americans do not have a non-English mother tongue accent, we also include an indicator for whether the respondent completed the interview in the Spanish language, with the expectation that this indicator is a proxy for those who are most sensitive that their identity as immigrants will be exposed, or sensitive that others will assume they are immigrants. We use an item that asks respondents how many times they visited their primary care doctors or clinics in the past year. The specific survey question asks: "Thinking about all of the members of your household, including adults and dependent children, approximately how many visits to primary care doctors or clinics have been made in the past year?" Given the question's wording and variability in household composition, we standardize this variable with the total number of individuals in the household with the following survey item, "What is the total number of persons living in your household?" We anticipate that frequency of contact with health care professionals, on average, is negatively associated with a skeptical view, suggesting either a continuation of safe encounters, or a "selection out" of people who have been adversely affected or want to preempt adverse consequences. Studies of distinct, but related, matters about social trust and trust in government suggest a generally positive relationship between age and trust, even considering period and cohort (Jennings and Stoker 2004; Robinson and Jackson 2001; Sutter and Kocher 2007). Our cross-sectional data limit our ability to disentangle age from period and cohort effects; however, we can include a measure of age in years. We also partial out a general sense of political sophistication and awareness about public policies using an eight-point ordinal scale of education level (1 = no formal schooling, 2 = Grades 1–8, 3 = some high school, 4 = high school diploma or GED, 5 = some college, 6 = Bachelor's Degree, 7 = Master's Degree, 8 = Doctoral level), and a four-point ordinal measure of whether a person pays attention to politics (0 = "hardly at all," 1 = "only now and then," 2 = "some of the time," 3 = "most of the time"). Finally, we also include an indicator for gender (1 if respondent identifies as a woman, 0 for man), to proxy for gender differences in health care experiences and caregiving responsibilities related to taking family members to see health care providers. Summary statistics for the variables used in this analysis are in table 2.

Our analytical approach here is to delve deeper into the link between immigration and health care. Latino US citizens are not the intended targets of restrictive immigration enforcement. However, we intend to evaluate the relationship between personal connections to those who are directly vulnerable to restrictive immigration enforcement and attitudes about the security of personal information that is shared in the context of a health clinic, health care provider's office, or hospital. The results of our regression analysis are reported in table 3. Statistical tests ($\beta = 0.407$; s.e. = 0.156) indicate that knowing someone who is undocumented is positively associated with the belief that personal information shared with health care providers is not secure (model 1). Similarly, knowing someone who has been deported ($\beta = 0.456$; s.e. = 0.152) is also associated with the skeptical view (model 2). These results are robust to alternative model specifications, including the inclusion and exclusion of alternative operationalizations of socioeconomic status indicators, the inclusion of state-fixed effects, and additional indicators for national origin.

To calculate the magnitude of the relationship, we can translate these logit model coefficients into predicted probabilities and relative risk figures. Visual evidence of the role of personal connections to undocumented and deported individuals is presented in figs. 3a–3d. The plots indicate

Table 2 Unweighted Summary Statistics of Covariates in Model of Attitude That Personal Information Shared with Health Care Providers Is Not Secure

Variable	N	Mean	Standard Deviation	Minimum	Maximum
Believes information is not secure	1,001	0.283	0.451	0	1
Knows someone who is undocumented	1,001	0.571	0.495	0	1
Knows someone who has been deported	1,001	0.411	0.492	0	1
Immigrant	1,001	0.248	0.432	0	1
Spanish-language interview	1,001	0.245	0.430	0	1
Mexican national origin	1,001	0.497	0.500	0	1
Doctor/clinic visits last year per family size	1,001	3.394	6.133	0	87
Highest education level completed	1,001	4.907	1.453	1	8
Income between $20,000 and $39,999	1,001	0.201	0.401	0	1
Income between $40,000 and $59,999	1,001	0.147	0.354	0	1
Income between $60,000 and $79,999	1,001	0.116	0.320	0	1
Income between $80,000 and $99,999	1,001	0.077	0.267	0	1
Income between $100,000 and $150,000	1,001	0.093	0.290	0	1
Income greater than $150,000	1,001	0.055	0.228	0	1
Income refused to report or missing	1,001	0.143	0.350	0	1
Woman	1,001	0.622	0.485	0	1
Attention to politics	1,001	2.898	1.037	1	4
Age in years	1,001	45	17.237	18	98

Source: 2015 Latino National Health and Immigration Survey.

that older age is positively correlated with skepticism about personal information ($\beta=0.010$; s.e. $=0.005$). For example, the upper-left panel traces the predicted probability of expressing skepticism about personal information being secure across the full range of age in years. The model predicts that people who know someone who is undocumented

Table 3   Logistic Regression of the Belief That Personal Information
Shared with Health Care Providers Is Not Secure, among Latino US Citizens

	Information Is Not Secure = 1	
	(1)	(2)
Knows someone who is undocumented	0.407*	
	(0.156)	
Knows someone who has been deported		0.456*
		(0.152)
Immigrant	−0.098	−0.080
	(0.184)	(0.184)
Spanish-language interview	−0.144	−0.095
	(0.200)	(0.198)
Mexican national origin	0.136	0.149
	(0.151)	(0.151)
Doctor/clinic visits last year per family size	−0.037	−0.038
	(0.020)	(0.021)
Highest education level completed	−0.084	−0.096
	(0.064)	(0.064)
Income between $20,000 and $39,999	−0.058	−0.054
	(0.249)	(0.249)
Income between $40,000 and $59,999	−0.263	−0.256
	(0.274)	(0.275)
Income between $60,000 and $79,999	0.245	0.274
	(0.290)	(0.290)
Income between $80,000 and $99,999	−0.567	−0.482
	(0.356)	(0.355)
Income between $100,000 and $150,000	0.131	0.210
	(0.322)	(0.323)
Income greater than $150,000	−0.439	−0.386
	(0.452)	(0.451)
Income refused to report or missing	0.009	0.017
	(0.261)	(0.261)
Woman	−0.451*	−0.427*
	(0.149)	(0.149)
Attention to politics	0.056	0.060
	(0.080)	(0.080)
Age in years	0.010*	0.011*
	(0.005)	(0.005)
Constant	−1.028*	−1.013*
	(0.426)	(0.423)
Observations	1,001	1,001
Log Likelihood	−536.980	−535.151
Akaike Inf. Crit.	1,107.960	1,104.301

Source: 2015 Latino National Health and Immigration Survey.
Note: Baseline for comparison of national origin indicators is "Mexico."
Baseline for comparison of income indicators is "less than $20,000."
*$p < 0.05$.

generally hold more skeptical views, no matter what their age. However, our ability to distinguish this difference or the actual relationship itself has considerable uncertainty as indicated by the overlapping 90 percent confidence bands across most ages. The exception is the estimate for individuals who are approximately 35 to 50 years of age, which includes the 45-year average age of respondents in our sample. The upper-right panel shows the model identifies distinctly greater skepticism among those who know someone who has been deported. Particularly for those people between the ages of 30 and 40, which coincides with the modal 30–39 years of age range of most deportees (TRAC 2014), the probability of expressing skepticism is estimated to be between 19 percent and 22 percent for someone who does not know someone who has been deported. By contrast, skepticism for this same age range is between 27 percent and 30 percent for people who do know someone who has been deported. The bottom panels translate this relationship into relative risks. Our statistical model estimates that a forty-five-year-old, the average age from our sample, who knows someone who is undocumented, is about 12 percent at greater risk of expressing a skeptical view regarding personal information shared with health care providers. For that same forty-five-year-old, knowing someone who has been deported corresponds to a 21 percent greater likelihood of being "at risk" of skepticism.

Also noteworthy, the number of doctor visits per household size is negatively associated with the skeptical view of personal information security. One possible explanation is that doctor visits provide greater exposure to health care providers, and this familiarity may reduce uncertainty about the systems and actors in health care settings. Experience with completing forms in a clinic setting and providing personal health information, particularly when it coincides with the absence of encounters with immigration authorities, may boost confidence that personal information is, in fact, secure in the hands of health care providers.

Similarly, women were less likely to express skeptical views. To the extent that women are generally more likely to handle health care appointments and visits for themselves and family members, this further corroborates the interpretation that repeat positive interactions facilitate familiarity and trust with health care-related organizations and actors. Another possibility is that because 85 percent of deportees are men (TRAC 2014), our model is picking up a broader skepticism that men hold in general about sharing personal information with any sources. Our data do not allow us to probe these explanations. However, the patterns in the relationships

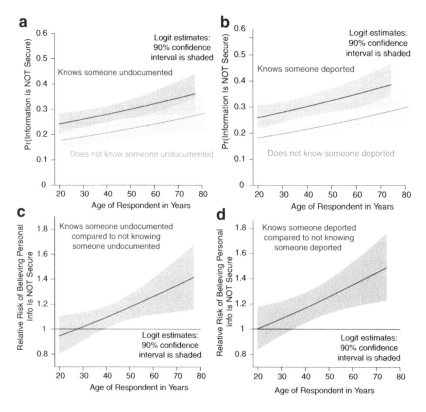

Figure 3a   The Relationship between Knowing Someone Who Is Undocumented and the Likelihood of Believing That Personal Information Shared with Health Care Providers Is Not Safe and Secure, across the Full Range of Values of Age in Years

Figure 3b   The Relationship between Knowing Someone Who Has Been Deported and the Likelihood of Believing That Personal Information Shared with Health Care Providers Is Not Safe and Secure, across the Full Range of Values of Age in Years

Figure 3c   The Relative Risk between Those Who Know Someone Who Is Undocumented and Those Who Do Not of Believing That Personal Information Shared with Health Care Providers Is Not Safe and Secure among, across the Full Range of Values of Age in Years

Figure 3d   The Relative Risk between Those Who Know Someone Who Has Been Deported and Those Who Do Not of Believing That Personal Information Shared with Health Care Providers Is Not Safe and Secure among, across the Full Range of Values of Age in Years

between skepticism of sharing personal information on the one hand, and personal connections as well as these demographic factors on the other, do lend support to the idea that restrictive immigration policy can induce people to shy away from health care-providing resources.

In a multivariate statistical model, we find no evidence of a relationship between either Spanish language interview or Mexican national heritage with the belief that personal information may be compromised in a health care setting. This non-finding may reflect the power of racial/ethnic profiling to influence the formation of attitudes for Latinos, in general.

Conclusion

On March 6, 2014, an interview with President Obama aired on Univision, a Spanish-language cable network, where he encouraged Latinos to sign up for health insurance using the online marketplace.[5] The appearance was part of a broader effort to secure the success of his marquee domestic policy, the ACA, which depended on a substantial number of uninsured individuals enrolling in a health insurance plan. President Obama explained that "part of the reason that it's so important for us to reach out to the Latino community is the Latino community is the most likely to be uninsured." For a brief moment, the interview became tense when Univision anchors played a video showing an undocumented woman who was afraid to enroll her US citizen children in a health insurance plan. She was concerned that immigration officials would use personal information collected through the online marketplace to deport her. President Obama assured the anchors and the audience that "none of the information that is provided in order for you to obtain health insurance is in any way transferred to immigration services." However, one observer remarked: "[Latino families] hear [the president's] assurance, but because of the level of deportations that have happened, there's a lot of families that don't know whether they can trust that assurance" (Easley 2014). For Latinos, the hyper-saliency of immigration trumps health and health care issues.

At the heart of President Obama's outreach campaign was a desire to reduce health care inequities. By expanding and subsidizing health insurance coverage, the ACA addressed cost as a major deterrent of access and use of health care services. However, the exchange above reveals another deterrent—widespread concern among Latinos about a general overlap

---

5. For the full transcript of the interview, see: www.communications-univisionnews.tumblr .com/post/79266471431/univision-news-transcript-interview-with.

between immigration policy and health care policy. While the concern may be concentrated among Latino immigrants, and especially undocumented immigrants, the woman's testimony indicates that Latino US citizens, in this case her children, are also stakeholders. The exchange also locates uncertainty about the connection between immigration and health care policies at points where personal information is shared in the course of applying for health care and social services. She did not use the language of policy feedback, but her worry suggests that she has internalized policy lessons that are similar to those learned by Latinos from past overlap between health, health care, and immigration policies. The implications for health care inequities are that, even if expansions and subsidies do their part to reduce costs, the politics of immigration may stymie engagement with health insurance marketplaces and the use of health care services in ways that are not presently addressed by health care reformers or health care management systems.

But, to what extent do these dynamics spill over to Latino US citizens? Our aim to assess the connection between the politics of immigration and use of health care resources began with an original, simple survey experiment. We extended our experimental analysis to compare the effects of immigration on engaging with other public services, and followed that up with a deeper dive into attitudes about the security of personal information that is shared with health care providers.

As we might expect from most exercises of this sort, the evidence is qualified. First, our experiment indicates a causal connection between the issue of immigration and the use of health care resources. By randomly assigning people to receive an "immigration issues" cue, we learned that Latino US citizens are nudged away from making appointments to see health care providers. Second, our subtle prime of immigration considerations continues to provoke an averse response, as indicated by a greater proportion of people who withhold from fully engaging in daily-life activities in order to avoid scrutiny of their citizenship status. The psychological aversion primed by "immigration issues" appears to operate to a greater extent for encounters with police, and to a lesser extent for encounters with educators. We view this as evidence that Latino US citizens practice cautious citizenship, and they do so broadly. Like previous studies, this one analysis suggests a broad effect of immigration policy, but it speaks less to whether these concerns about immigration are also related to what happens once people do make appointments to see a health care provider.

Police, educators, and health care providers are all examples of public servants who are difficult to interface with anonymously. This point motivated us to further interrogate the role of sharing personal information with health care providers. Our contribution on this front reveals the depth of the connection between immigration politics and health care. Skepticism about the security of personal information in the hands of doctors, nurses, and health care administrators is correlated with knowing someone who has been deported. Clearly, for some individuals the stakes may be revealing one's citizenship status to law enforcement officials, thus jeopardizing their unlawful residence in the United States. For others, it may be a move to protect family members who have an unauthorized presence in the United States, or to avoid family separation. Whatever the case, these indirect experiences with immigration enforcement parallel the reticence to engage with public programs and government that scholars in the policy feedback tradition anticipate and have found in other contexts. In this case, however, we see that public policy (immigration) appears to inform attitudes about professionals that are seemingly unrelated to that particular policy (health care providers), and it does so among people who are not supposed to be the direct targets of that policy. These results build on and extend considerably the literature regarding racial inequities in provider trust—one important factor that contributes to health and health care inequities. The findings from our investigation suggest that racializing policies shift the propensity for Latino US citizens to make an appointment to see a health care provider, and proximity to undocumented immigrants shapes their concerns that information shared with health care providers is not secure.

Yet, the subtle cue in our experiment does not fully capture the range of existing immigration policy. Our strategy fulfilled our purpose to test the "balance" of considerations that would be cued by the phrase "immigration issues." Documenting the causal effects of explicitly expansive and explicitly restrictive immigration policy is an exercise for future experimental analysis. Although our experiment takes place over the course of a telephone or Web-based interview, analogous field experiments may present themselves as national and sub-national immigrant policy shifts. Whatever the direction that immigration politics takes, it is very likely that immigration will remain a highly salient issue for Latinos. In 2017, President Obama's successor entered the White House after a campaign of promises for more restrictive immigration policy, suggesting that the dynamics identified in this study will remain relevant to the provision of health care, and, by extension, to the study of health and health care inequities.

The statistical results suggest that skepticism about the security of personal information shared with health care providers is about more than just a general distrust of health care practitioners. The correlation to knowing someone who has been deported fits the narrative that at least some Latinos live by a calculus to manage the risk of exposing one's citizenship status. Still, our analysis does not rule out the possibility that the mechanism through which distrust develops is the performance of health care providers. Nevertheless, for many such practitioners, Latinos represent a growing share of their patient roster. And, from what we learned in this investigation, the salience of immigration follows people into their interactions with health care practitioners. If trust in health care providers corrodes in response to linkages with immigration policy, then where does that leave doctors, nurses, health care administrators, and others who are taking on the mission to reduce health care inequities?

One strategy that health care providers can adopt is to provide all patients with assurances at the point of intake that their personal information is kept private and secure, and to implement policies and practices that support this assurance. To the extent that this is a promise that they can keep, they should announce this commitment broadly and frequently. A second strategy is to coordinate this commitment with other organizations and services such as local immigrant advocacy organizations and local police whose job may also be hampered by spillover from immigration politics. In some ways doctors are like police: both solve puzzles that involve humans in need of help, and their successes are shaped by the extent to which individuals and communities trust them and their institutions. Perhaps doctors can learn from local law enforcement agencies that have experience dealing with publics that are reluctant to call them for services or disclose information that helps them do their job. A third strategy is to "go public" with the issue. Health care providers are represented by various interest groups and associations, such as the American Medical Association and American Nurses Association, and elected officials are attentive to constituent concerns, especially those that are coordinated and persistent. If the politics of immigration is keeping Latinos from seeing their doctors and nurses, or discouraging Latinos from providing all the information that is needed to assign appropriate diagnoses and treatments, then doctors are stakeholders in immigration policy. By introducing such complications to the provision of health care, we suspect that the politics of immigration injects a new source of inefficiency and greater costs associated with delayed treatment. For these reasons, the political arena may be a fruitful place for doctors and nurses to explain that immigration enforcement is interfering with their ability to deliver services, and makes the services they do deliver more expensive.

A central challenge of efforts to achieve health equity is that many of the organizations and policies that address health care-related issues operate in a broader institutional and policy context. This investigation joins a growing number of studies that are uncovering how immigration policy is health care policy. Any effort to address health care inequities is impeded by a lack of understanding of how contemporary immigration politics conditions people to stay away from, or distrust interactions with, health care providers.

■ ■ ■

Francisco I. Pedraza is assistant professor of political Science in the School of Public Policy at University of California, Riverside. Professor Pedraza is an alumnus (Cohort 19, 2012–14) of the RWJF Scholars in Health Policy Research Program. He served as co-principal investigator on the 2015 Latino National Health and Immigration Survey. His research focuses broadly on explaining the political attitudes and behavior of Latinos and other minority groups and immigrants in the United States. fpedraza@ucr.edu

Vanessa Cruz Nichols is a PhD candidate in political science at the University of Michigan. Vanessa's research interests include Latino politics, race and ethnicity politics, political participation, public opinion, and identity politics. She has received support to conduct research from the Ford Foundation as a predoctoral and dissertation fellow, and from the National Science Foundation Doctoral Dissertation Research Improvement Grant. Vanessa's dissertation, "Latinos Rising to the Challenge: Political Responses to Threat and Opportunity Messages," focuses on mobilizing messages and how they might create a more engaged or disengaged citizenry. Vanessa is a co-student investigator with the 2015 Latino National Health and Immigrant Survey.

Alana M. W. LeBrón is assistant professor of public health and Chicano/Latino studies at University of California, Irvine. Her research focuses broadly on the contributions of social inequalities to inequities in health for Latina/o communities, and the intersections of race, class, gender, and immigration-related factors on these processes.

Acknowledgments

We gratefully acknowledge the helpful comments of Claire Adida, Matt Barreto, Dan Biggers, Alan Cohen, Loren Collingwood, Kim Yi Dionne, Mary Waters, Laura Evans, Colleen Grogan, Jed Horwitt, Tiffany Joseph, Julia Lynch, Silvia Manzano, Jamila Michener, Rashawn Ray, Gabriel Sanchez, Abigail A. Sewell, Edward Vargas, Omar Wasow, Mary Waters, Jessie Wolf, and Jessica Yen.

References

Barreto, Matt A., and Gary M. Segura. 2010. "Latino Voters Strongly Reject Arizona Immigration Law 1070." *Latino Decisions*, www.latinodecisions.com/blog/2010/05/06/latino-voters-strongly-reject-arizona-immigration-law-1070/.

Beniflah, Jacob D., Wendalyn K. Little, Harold K. Simon, and Jesse Sturm. 2013. "Effects of Immigration Enforcement Legislation on Hispanic Pediatric Patient Visits to the Pediatric Emergency Department." *Clinical Pediatrics* 52, no. 12: 1122–26.

Burch, Traci. 2013. *Trading Democracy for Justice: Criminal Convictions and the Decline of Neighborhood Political Participation*. Chicago: University of Chicago Press.

Campbell, Andrea L. 2002. "Self-Interest, Social Security, and the Distinctive Participation Patterns of Senior Citizens." *American Political Science Review* 96, no. 3: 565–74.

Campbell, Andrea L. 2007. "Universalism, Targeting, and Participation." In *Remaking America: Democracy and Public Policy in an Age of Inequality*, edited by Joe Soss, Jacobs S. Hacker, and Suzanne Mettler, 121–40. New York: Russell Sage Foundation.

Castañeda, Heide, and Milena A. Melo. 2014. "Health Care Access for Latino Mixed-Status Families: Barriers, Strategies, and Implications for Reform." *American Behavioral Scientist* 58, no. 14: 1891–1909.

Cavazos-Rehg, Patricia A., Luis H. Zayas, and Edward L. Spitznagel. 2007. "Legal Status, Emotional Well-Being and Subjective Health Status of Latino Immigrants." *Journal of the National Medical Association* 99, no. 10: 1126–31.

Chavez, Leo R. 2008. *The Latino Threat*. Stanford, CA: Stanford University Press.

Chin, Marshall H., Ame E. Walters, Scott C. Cook, and Elbert S. Huang. 2007. "Interventions to Reduce Racial and Ethnic Disparities in Health Care." *Medical Care Research and Review* 64, Supplement 5: S7–S28.

Converse, Phillip E. 1964. "The Nature of Belief Systems in Mass Publics." In *Ideology and Discontent*, edited by David E. Apter, 206–61. New York: Free Press.

Cox, Adam B., and Thomas J. Miles. 2013. "Policing Immigration." *University of Chicago Law Review* 80, no. 1: 87–136.

Daniels, Roger. 2005. *Guarding the Golden Door*. New York: Hill and Wang.

DeRose, Kathryn Pitkin, Jose J. Escarce, and Nicole Lurie. 2007. "Immigrants and Health Care: Sources of Vulnerability." *Health Affairs* 26, no. 5: 1258–68.

Donelson, Katelynn. 2015. "Medical Repatriation: The Dangerous Intersection of Health Care Law and Immigration." *Journal of Health Care Law and Policy* 18, no. 2: 347–69.

Easley, Jonathan. 2014. "Obama to Hispanics: We Won't Deport Relatives Because You Enroll in Obamacare." *The Hill*, www.thehill.com/policy/healthcare/201076 -obama-makes-o-care-pitch-to-hispanics-the.

Fiske, Susan T., and Shelley E. Taylor. 1991. *Social Cognition*. New York: McGraw-Hill.

Fix, Michael E., and Jeffery S. Passel. 1999. "Trends in Non-Citizens' and Citizens' Use of Public Benefits Following Welfare Reform: 1994–1997." Washington, DC: Urban Institute.

Fox, Cybelle. 2012. *Three Words of Relief: Race, Immigration and the American Welfare State from the Progressive Era to the New Deal*. Princeton, NJ: Princeton University Press.

Fox, Cybelle. 2016. "Unauthorized Welfare: The Origins of Immigrant Status Restrictions in American Social Policy." *Journal of American History* 102, no. 4: 1051–74.

Fraga, Luis R., Rodney E. Hero, John A. Garcia, Michael Jones-Correa, Val Martinez-Ebers, and Gary M. Segura. 2011. *Latinos in the New Millennium: An Almanac of Opinion, Behavior, and Policy Preferences*. New York: Cambridge University Press.

Gee, Gilbert C., and Chandra L. Ford. 2011. "Structural Racism and Health Inequities: Old Issues, New Directions." *DuBois Review* 8, no. 1: 115–32.

Golash-Boza, Tanya Maria. 2012. *Immigration Nation: Raids, Detentions, and Deportation in Post-9/11 America*. Boulder, CO: Paradigm Publishers.

Gratton, Brian, and Emily Klancher Merchant. 2015. "An Immigrant's Tale: The Mexican American Southwest, 1850 to 1950." *Social Science History* 39, no. 4: 521–50.

Gutiérrez, David A., ed. 2004. *The Columbia History of Latinos in the United States Since 1960*. New York: Columbia University Press.

Hacker, Karen, Jocelyn Chu, Carolyn Leung, Robert Marra, Alex Pirie, Mohamed Brahimi, Margaret English, Joshua Beckmann, Dolores Acevedo-Garcia, and Robert P. Marlin. 2011. "The Impact of Immigration and Customs Enforcement on Immigrant Health: Perceptions of Immigrants in Everett, Massachusetts, USA." *Social Science and Medicine* 73, no. 4: 586–94.

Hutchings, Vincent L. 2003. *Public Opinion and Democratic Accountability: How Citizens Learn about Politics*. Princeton, NJ: Princeton University Press.

Jacobson, Robin. 2008. *The New Nativism: Proposition 187 and the Debate over Immigration*. Minneapolis: University of Minnesota Press.

Jennings, M. Kent, and Laura Stoker. 2004. "Social Trust and Civic Engagement across Time and Generations." *Acta Politica* 39, no. 4: 342–79.

Jiménez, Tomás R. 2008. "Mexican Immigrant Replenishment and the Continuing Significance of Ethnicity and Race." *American Journal of Sociology* 113, no. 6: 1527–67.

Joseph, Tiffany D. 2016. "What Healthcare Reform Means for Immigrants: A Comparison of the Affordable Care Act and Massachusetts Health Reform." *Journal of Health Politics, Policy, and Law* 41, no. 1: 101–16.

Kalet, Hank. 2009. "Undocumented Immigrants Living in the Shadows." Online, centraljersey.com, "Dispatches," May 26. www.centraljersey.com/opinion/dispatches -undocumented-immigrants-living-in-the-shadows/article_729df788-fe50-5b48-a297 -4f86f4ac823c.html.

Karpman, Michael, and Sharon K. Long. 2015. "Taking Stock: Gains in Health Insurance Coverage under the ACA Continue as of September 2015, but Many Remain Uninsured." Urban Institute Health Policy Center, www.hrms.urban.org /quicktakes/Gains-in-Health-Insurance-Coverage-under-the-ACA-Continue-as-of -September-2015-but-Many-Remain-Uninsured.html.

Key, Valdimer O. 1966. *The Responsible Electorate: Rationality in Presidential Voting, 1936–1960.* Cambridge, MA: Belknap Press of Harvard University.

Kilbourne, Amy M., Galen Switzer, Kelly Hyman, Megan Crowley-Matoka, and Michael J. Fine. 2008. "Advancing Health Disparities Research within the Health Care System." *American Journal of Public Health* 96: 2113–21.

Kohli, Aarti, and Lisa Chavez. 2013. "The Federal Secure Communities Program and Young Men of Color in California." Chief Justice Earl Warren Institute on Law and Social Policy. www.law.berkeley.edu/files/BMOC_Secure_Communities_Program_ FINAL.pdf.

Koulish, Robert E. 2010. *Immigration and American Democracy: Subverting the Rule of Law.* New York: Routledge.

Krosnick, Jon A. 1990. "Government Policy and Citizen Passion: A Study of Issue Publics in Contemporary America." *Political Behavior* 12, no. 1: 59–92.

Lopez, Mark Hugo, Ana Gonzalez-Barrera, and Jens Manuel Krogstad. 2014. "Latino Support for Democrats Falls, but Democratic Advantage Remains: Immigration Not a Deal-breaker Issue for Half of Latino Voters." Washington, DC: Pew Research Center. www.pewhispanic.org/files/2014/10/2014-10-29_NSL-latino -politics.pdf.

Manzano, Sylvia. 2011. "One Year After S. B. 1070: Why Immigration Will Not Go Away." *Latino Decisions,* www.latinodecisions.com/blog/2011/05/09/one-year -after-sb1070-why-immigration-will-not-go-away/.

Massey, Douglas S. 2002. *Beyond Smoke and Mirrors: Mexican Immigration in an Era of Economic Integration.* New York: Russell Sage Foundation.

Massey, Douglas S. 2013. "Immigration as a Race-Making Institution." In *Immigration, Poverty, and Socioeconomic Inequality,* edited by David Card and Steven Raphael, 257–81. New York: Russell Sage Foundation.

Meissner, Doris, Donald M. Kerwin, Muzaffar Chishti, and Claire Bergeron. 2013. "Immigration Enforcement in the United States: The Rise of a Formidable Machinery." Migration Policy Institute Technical Report.

Mettler, Suzanne. 2005. *Soldiers to Citizens.* New York: Oxford University Press.

Minkler, Meredith. 2010. "Linking Science and Policy through Community-Based Participatory Research to Study and Address Health Disparities." *American Journal of Public Health* Supplement 1: S81–S87.

Miranda, Patricia Y., Amy J. Schulz, Barbara A. Israel, and Hector M. González. 2011. "Context of Entry and Number of Depressive Symptoms in an Older Mexican-Origin Immigrant Population." *Journal of Immigrant and Minority Health* 13, no. 4: 706–12.

Molina, Natalia. 2006. *Fit to Be Citizens? Public Health and Race in Los Angeles, 1879–1939.* Stanford, CA: Stanford University Press.

Mutz, Diana C. 2011. *Population-Based Survey Experiments.* Princeton, NJ: Princeton University Press.

Myers, Dowell. 2007. *Immigrants and Boomers: Forging a New Social Contract for the Future of America.* New York: Russell Sage Foundation.

National Council of La Raza. 2014. "Immigration is Personal to Latino Voters." *Huffington Post*, blog, www.huffingtonpost.com/national-council-of-la-raza-/immigration-is-personal-t_b_5998666.html.

Ngai, Mae M. 2004. *Impossible Subjects: Illegal Aliens and the Making of Modern America.* Princeton, NJ: Princeton University Press.

Nicholson, Stephen P. 2005. *Voting the Agenda: Candidates, Elections, and Ballot Propositions.* Princeton, NJ: Princeton University Press.

Park, Lisa. 2011. *Entitled to Nothing: The Struggle for Immigrant Health Care in the Age of Welfare Reform.* New York: New York University Press.

PBS (Public Broadcasting Service). 2011. "Why Three Governors Challenged Secure Communities." *Frontline.* www.pbs.org/wgbh/pages/frontline/race-multicultural/lost-in-detention/why-three-governors-challenged-secure-communities/.

Pedroza, Juan Manuel. 2013. "Removal Roulette: Secure Communities and Immigration Enforcement in the United States." In *Outside Justice: Immigration and the Criminalizing Impact of Changing Policy and Practice*, edited by David C. Brotherton, Daniel L. Stageman, and Shirley P. Leyro, 45–65. New York: Springer.

Pew Hispanic Center. 2007. "2007 National Survey of Latinos: As Illegal Immigration Issue Heats Up, Hispanics Feel a Chill." Washington, DC: Pew Hispanic Center, www.pewhispanic.org/2007/12/13/2007-national-survey-of-latinos-as-illegal-immigration-issue-heats-up-hispanics-feel-a-chill/.

Pierson, Paul. 1993. "When Effects Become Causes: Policy Feedback and Policy Changes." *World Politics* 45, no. 4: 595–628.

Raymond-Flesch, Marissa, Rachel Siemons, Nadereh Pourat, Ken Jacobs, and Claire D. Brindis. 2014. "'There Is No Help Out There and If There Is, It's Really Hard to Find': A Qualitative Study of the Health Concerns and Health Care Access of Latino 'DREAMers.'" *Journal of Adolescent Health*, 55: 323–28.

Reverby, Susan M. 2011. "'Normal Exposure' and Inoculation Syphilis: A PHS 'Tuskegee' Doctor in Guatemala, 1946–48." *Journal of Policy History* 23: 6–28.

Rhodes, Scott D., Lilli Mann, Florence M. Simán, Eunyoung Song, Jorge Alonzo, Mario Downs, Emma Lawlor et al. 2015. "The Impact of Local Immigration Enforcement Policies on the Health of Immigrant Hispanics/Latinos in the United States." *American Journal of Public Health* 105, no. 2: 329–37.

Robinson, Robert V., and Elton F. Jackson. 2001. "Is Trust in Others Declining in America? An Age-Period-Cohort Analysis." *Social Science Research* 30, no. 1: 117–45.

Rocha, Rene R., Benjamin R. Knoll, and Robert D. Wrinkle. 2015. "Immigration Enforcement and the Redistribution of Political Trust." *Journal of Politics* 77, no. 4: 901–13.

Rosenstone, Steven J., and John Mark Hansen. 1993. *Mobilization, Participation, and Democracy in America*. London: Longman.

Sampaio, Anna. 2015. *Terrorizing Latina/o Immigrants: Race, Gender, and Immigration Policy Post-9/11*. Philadelphia: Temple University Press.

Schneider, Anne, and Helen Ingram. 1993. "Social Construction of Target Populations." *American Political Science Review* 87, no. 2: 334–47.

Sewell, Abigail A. 2015. "Disaggregating Ethnoracial Disparities in Physician Trust." *Social Science Research*, 54: 1–20.

Smedley, Brian D., Adrienne Y. Stith, and Alan R. Nelson. 2003. *Unequal Treatment: Confronting Racial and Ethnic Disparities in Health Care*. Washington, DC: National Academy.

Soss, Joe. 2002. *Unwanted Claims: The Politics of Participation in the U.S. Welfare System*. Ann Arbor: University of Michigan Press.

Stern, Alexandra M., Nicole L. Novak, Natalie Lira, Kate O'Connor, Siobán Harlow, and Sharon Kardia. 2017. "California's Sterilization Survivors: An Estimate and Call for Redress." *American Journal of Public Health*, 107: 50–54.

Sutter, Matthias, and Martin G. Kocher. 2007. "Trust and Trustworthiness across Different Age Groups." *Games and Economic Behavior* 59, no. 2: 364–82.

Taylor, Shelley E., and Susan T. Fiske. 1978. "Salience, Attention, and Attribution: Top of the Head Phenomena." In *Advances in Social Psychology*, edited by Leonard Berkowitz, 249–88. New York: Academic.

Toomey, Russell B., A. J. Umana-Taylor, David R. Williams, Elizabeth Harvey-Mendoza, Laudan B. Jahromi, and Kimberly A. Updegraff. 2014. "Impact of Arizona's S. B. 1070 Immigration Law on Utilization of Health Care and Public Assistance among Mexican-Origin Adolescent Mothers and their Mother Figures." *American Journal of Public Health* 104, no. S1: S28–S34.

TRAC (Transactional Records Access Clearinghouse). 2014. "ICE Deportations: Gender, Age, and Country of Citizenship." Transactional Records Access Clearinghouse, www.trac.syr.edu/immigration/reports/350/.

Vallejo, Laura. 2010. "Catholic Immigrants Frightened by the List." *Intermountain Catholic*, www.icatholic.org/article/catholic-immigrants-frightened-by-the-list-965612.

Vargas, Edward D. 2015. "Immigration Enforcement and Mixed-Status Families: The Effect of Risk of Deportation on Medicaid Use." *Children Youth Services Review* 57: 83–89.

Verba, Sidney, Kay Lehman Schlozman, and Henry Brady. 1995. *Voice and Equality: Civic Voluntarism in American Politics*. Cambridge, MA: Harvard University Press.

Viruell-Fuentes, Edna A., Patricia Y. Miranda, and Sawsan Abdulrahim. 2012. "More Than Culture: Structural Racism, Intersectionality Theory, and Immigrant Health." *Social Science and Medicine* 75, no. 12: 2099–2106.

Walker, Hannah L. 2014. "Extending the Effects of the Carceral State: Proximal Contact, Political Participation and Race." *Political Research Quarterly* 67, no. 4: 809–22.

Watson, Tara. 2014. "Inside the Refrigerator: Immigration Enforcement and Chilling Effects in Medicaid Participation." *American Economic Journal: Economic Policy* 6, no. 3: 313–38.

Weaver, Vesla M., and Amy E. Lerman. 2010. "Political Consequences of the Carceral State." *American Political Science Review* 104, no. 4: 817–33.

Welch, Michael. 2002. *Detained: Immigration Laws and the Expanding I.N.S. Jail Complex*. Philadelphia: Temple University Press.

Zayas, Luis. 2015. *Forgotten Citizen: Deportation, Children, and the Making of American Exiles and Orphans*. Oxford: Oxford University Press.

Zimmermann, Wendy, and Michael Fix. 1998. "Declining Immigrant Applications for Medical and Welfare Benefits in Los Angeles County." Washington, DC: Urban Institute.

Falling through the Coverage Cracks: How Documentation Status Minimizes Immigrants' Access to Health Care

Tiffany D. Joseph
Stony Brook University

Abstract Recent policy debates have centered on health reform and who should benefit from such policy. Most immigrants are excluded from the 2010 Affordable Care Act (ACA) due to federal restrictions on public benefits for certain immigrants. But, some subnational jurisdictions have extended coverage options to federally ineligible immigrants. Yet, less is known about the effectiveness of such inclusive reforms for providing coverage and care to immigrants in those jurisdictions. This article examines the relationship between coverage and health care access for immigrants under comprehensive health reform in the Boston metropolitan area. The article uses data from interviews conducted with a total of 153 immigrants, health care professionals, and immigrant and health advocacy organization employees under the Massachusetts and ACA health reforms. Findings indicate that respondents across the various stakeholder groups perceive that immigrants' documentation status minimizes their ability to access health care even when they have health coverage. Specifically, respondents expressed that intersecting public policies, concerns that using health services would jeopardize future legalization proceedings, and immigrants' increased likelihood of deportation en route to medical appointments negatively influenced immigrants' health care access. Thus, restrictive federal policies and national-level anti-immigrant sentiment can undermine inclusive subnational policies in socially progressive places.

Keywords health policy, immigrants, Chapter 58

Funding for this project was provided by the American Sociological Association Funding Across the Discipline Program, Robert Wood Johnson Foundation Health Policy Scholars Program, and Woodrow Wilson Foundation.

Journal of Health Politics, Policy and Law, Vol. 42, No. 5, October 2017
DOI 10.1215/03616878-3940495   © 2017 by Duke University Press

Introduction

Recent policy debates have centered on health reform, who should benefit from such policy, and, to what extent, if any, immigrants (especially the unauthorized) should be included in comprehensive health reform. Given federal restrictions to public benefits for certain immigrants, most are excluded from provisions of the 2010 Affordable Care Act (ACA). Yet, some subnational jurisdictions (e.g., Massachusetts) have extended coverage options to federally ineligible immigrants (Joseph 2016). Much less is known, however, about how effective these inclusive health reforms have been in providing coverage and care to eligible immigrants in those jurisdictions. Since previous studies have shown that increasing access to coverage does not guarantee increased use of health services, it is important to understand what factors influence individuals' health service use, particularly when they have coverage.

This article explores the relationship between coverage and health care access for immigrants under health reform, with specific attention to how documentation status presents various challenges to care for this group. Specifically, this article illustrates how health policy's intersection with other types of public policy (e.g., welfare, driving) amid increasing anti-immigrant sentiment influences immigrants' health care decisions. Cumulatively, these sociopolitical dynamics undermine health equity attempts for noncitizens, who comprise 13 percent of the US population. As few studies have qualitatively examined immigrants' health care experiences under state and federal health reform, this article will help researchers, policy makers, and the general public better understand how documentation status and public policy facilitate social inequality in the health care system.

Literature Review

Immigrants' Exclusion in Public Policy

Existing public policy has significantly limited most immigrants'—undocumented and documented—access to various services in recent decades (Fox 2016; Joseph 2016; Park 2011). Notably, the 1996 Illegal Immigration Reform and Immigrant Responsibility Act (IIRIRA) and the 1996 Personal Responsibility and Work Opportunity Act (PRWORA) made immigrants of any documentation status more susceptible to deportation and reduced their access to public benefits (Fox 2016; Park 2011). The IIRIRA increased border security, criminalized falsified immigration documents, and verified employment eligibility (IIRIRA 1996). The PRWORA applied a five-year residency bar for eligibility for public benefits for legal permanent residents (LPRs, or green card holders) (Fox 2016). This also meant that unauthorized immigrants and visa holders became federally ineligible for public benefits (Capps and Fix 2013; Fox 2016).[1] But, states could extend benefits to ineligible immigrants by using state funds and passing legislation for this purpose (Warner 2012). The present-day enforcement of these policies alongside anti-immigrant attitudes generates ongoing exclusion for immigrants (Fox 2016; Marrow and Joseph 2015).

With no comprehensive federal immigration reform since IIRIRA, immigrants are unable to regularize their status. In this absence, presidential executive orders and state-level policies have been created. Former president Obama's 2012 Deferred Action for Childhood Arrivals (DACA) program granted temporary relief from deportation, and work authorization and driver's licenses (in some states) to unauthorized young adults brought to the United States as children.[2] Forty-six states have also passed laws granting or restricting unauthorized immigrants from receiving state-funded public benefits or obtaining housing (Ybarra, Sanchez, and Sanchez 2015).

The Massachusetts and Affordable Care Act Health Reforms

Although the ACA was signed into law in 2010, the policy was modeled after the 2006 Massachusetts health reform known as Chapter 58 (Joseph 2016; Patel and McDonough 2010). Unlike the ACA, Massachusetts included provisions for income-eligible state residents of any documentation status through the Health Safety Net (HSN) and Commonwealth Care (CommCare) programs.[3] Unauthorized immigrants could also directly purchase coverage in the state's health insurance exchange. Some immigrants may likely have had coverage from their employers or spouses.

Because of Massachusetts' compliance with the ACA, state lawmakers prepared for full ACA implementation in October 2013. Lawmakers recrafted the original Chapter 58 reform to maintain coverage for federally

1. Immigrants with temporary protected status (TPS, or refugee/asylee) can receive public benefits their first seven years in the country.
2. DACA does not provide LPR status and is not a path to citizenship (Batalova et al. 2013). As DACA is an executive order that President Trump and many Republicans oppose, this program (and associated benefits) for DACA recipients may end under Trump's administration.
3. See Joseph (2016) for income-level cutoffs and eligibility for immigrant groups under Chapter 58 and the ACA.

ineligible immigrants. Since HSN and CommCare were state-funded, these programs were not changed substantially immediately after ACA implementation.[4] But, unauthorized immigrants lost their ability to purchase coverage in the Massachusetts exchange under the ACA.

Nationally, under the ACA (in compliant states), only adult US citizens, long-term LPRs, and TPS immigrants were eligible for provisions through the Medicaid expansion or participation in the health exchanges (Capps and Fix 2013; Marrow and Joseph 2015). Most noncitizens' federal ineligibility for ACA provisions stemmed from the PRWORA and IIRIRA policies.[5] Visa holders and income-eligible short-term LPRs could purchase coverage in the exchanges, but undocumented immigrants could not (Joseph 2016). Most immigrants' exclusion from the ACA meant that many remained uninsured (Capps and Fix 2013). Their main option for obtaining health services was in safety net hospitals and clinics, which received fewer funds for indigent health care costs under the ACA as more Americans theoretically obtained coverage (Portes, Fernández-Kelly, and Light 2012). Conversely, the ACA increased federal funding by $22 billion over five fiscal years to Federally Qualified Health Centers (FQHCs), which provide primary care and some specialty care to medically underserved populations (Patel and McDonough 2010). This might have been the only way federally ineligible immigrants could access health services under the policy (Warner 2012).

Ineligible immigrants' lack of access to federally subsidized health care has also yielded an increase in medical repatriations—"the process by which uninsured aliens who suffer from long-term medical care needs are transferred from a United States hospital to a medical care facility in their country of origin" (Donelson 2015: 348; Zoellner 2010). While exact numbers are unknown, estimates suggest that 800 medical deportations occurred in the years 2006–2012 across 15 states (NYLPI 2012; Schumann 2016). These deportations typically happen because hospitals do not receive federal reimbursement for providing nonemergency care to indigent

4. CommCare underwent a name change to ConnectorCare. Funding for HSN has been reduced significantly. On June 1, 2016, HSN income eligibility was reduced from 400 percent FPL to 300 percent FPL, the retroactive eligibility period was reduced from 6 months to 10 days, and deductibles were implemented for HSN patients with incomes of 150 percent FPL and above (Mass.gov 2016; Mass Legal Services 2016). Local health advocacy and immigrant organizations are concerned these changes will negatively affect HSN recipients' health care access, especially federally ineligible immigrants with no other coverage options given their exclusion from the ACA.

5. Low-income DACA recipients under age 18 are eligible for ACA coverage through the Children's Health Insurance Program (CHIP). This may change pending President Trump's anti-immigrant stance and anticipated repeal of the ACA.

immigrant patients (Zoellner 2010). It is likely medical repatriations will increase among immigrants amid their exclusion from ACA provisions and other public benefits.

When comparing the Massachusetts and ACA reforms, Massachusetts immigrants have access to greater coverage relative to immigrants elsewhere nationwide (Joseph 2016).[6] While increased inclusive health coverage reduced the state's uninsured population to 3.1 percent by 2011, this percentage did not include federally ineligible immigrants (Long, Goin, and Lynch 2013).[7] After ACA implementation, the state's uninsurance level fluctuated between 3.1 and 4.0 percent during 2011–2015, remaining the nation's lowest (Chin et al. 2016).[8] But, it is estimated that more than 200,000 residents—low income, Hispanic, young adult, and male—remained uninsured due to being unable to afford coverage, being unaware of how to obtain coverage, becoming unemployed or changing employers, or losing eligibility for public coverage (Chin et al. 2016). Coverage options are also delineated by documentation status, and patients with publicly subsidized coverage (federal or state) experience greater difficulty using it, as physicians can opt out of serving patients with such plans (Decker 2012). In the best-case scenario of Massachusetts, one's documentation status (and income) facilitate differences in health care even *with* coverage.

Pre- and Post-Reform Health Care Barriers for Immigrants

Prior to PRWORA, IIRIRA, and the ACA, federally ineligible immigrants could access health services by obtaining private insurance (on their own or via their own or a spouse's employer), or by receiving required treatment to stabilize severe conditions in the emergency department (Warner 2012).[9] Certain vulnerable populations (e.g., pregnant women, children) could access subsidized care via specific Medicaid programs (Marrow 2012; Warner 2012). However, despite their previous less generous access to health services, noncitizens of different documentation statuses utilize these services less frequently than citizens even when they have coverage (Tarraf, Vega, and González 2014).

6. See Marrow and Joseph (2015) for more on immigrants' coverage options in other states that have extended coverage to federally ineligible immigrants.
7. Data on the state's public coverage options do not include usage statistics by documentation status (Joseph 2016).
8. Some of this fluctuation was likely due to the MA-ACA transition in which some residents became uninsured when the state's online exchange failed (Cheney 2014; McDonough 2016).
9. The 1986 Emergency Medical Treatment and Labor Act (EMTALA) requires hospitals receiving federal funds to treat emergency department patients regardless of their ability to pay.

Under the ACA, intensified anti-immigrant sentiment in public policy and among the general population has had a profound chilling effect on immigrants' health care access (see Pedraza, this volume). Documentation status concerns for immigrants themselves or family members present a significant barrier to health care access (Fox 2016; Joseph 2016). Documented immigrants, particularly in mixed-status families, may be less likely to use eligible health services out of fear that their naturalization or that of family members will be jeopardized (Park 2011). Using such services may also draw attention to unauthorized relatives, increasing their chances for detention and/or deportation (Castañeda and Melo 2014).

Additionally, lack of English proficiency and provider-patient cultural concordance also limit immigrants' (and some citizens') health care access, yielding lower quality of care and misdiagnoses for minority and immigrant patients (Betancourt and Bondaryk 2014; IOM 2002; Sentell and Braun 2012). While the nation has become more diverse, such diversity is not reflected among predominantly white health care providers (HHS 2015). Societal implicit biases toward minority groups may also inadvertently lead to discrimination in the health care system (Betancourt and Bondaryk 2014; IOM 2002; Shavers et al. 2012).

Finally, complex bureaucratic (re)enrollment procedures constrain immigrants' health care access (López-Sanders 2013; Marrow 2012). Inability to complete health coverage forms available only in English or Spanish, or produce income eligibility information, bureaucratically disentitles immigrants from applying for benefits for which they are eligible (Marrow 2012; Marrow and Joseph 2015). Relatedly, immigrants' lack of literacy of the complex US health care system (i.e., primary versus specialty care) limits their ability to adequately use health services when they have coverage (Tarraf, Vega, and González 2014).

Much of what researchers know about immigrants' health care coverage and access is based on quantitative studies conducted before the implementation of comprehensive federal health reform. However, because immigrants, especially the unauthorized, are difficult to access, quantitative studies are limited in their ability to provide a comprehensive analysis of this population. Thus, small-scale qualitative studies have provided significant insight into the health care challenges immigrants face (Hacker et al. 2012; López-Sanders 2013; Marrow 2012). But, since ACA implementation, few studies have qualitatively explored how changing health and other types of public policy are reshaping immigrants' health care access (Chin et al. 2016). The pre- and post-ACA qualitative assessment of Boston immigrants' health care experiences in this article will make a significant contribution, enhancing researchers and policy makers' understanding of how macro-level health policy is affecting this population at the micro level.

Methods

Data for this study were obtained from a larger investigation examining how being an immigrant shaped one's qualitative experiences with the health care system from 2012 to 2013 (under Chapter 58) and 2015 to 2016 (after ACA implementation) in Boston, Massachusetts.[10] To assess the influence of comprehensive health reform (pre- and post-ACA implementation) for immigrants, a total of 153 individuals were interviewed, comprising three stakeholder groups: immigrants, health care professionals, and immigrant and health advocacy organization employees. Table 1 shows the composition of the 2012–13 and 2015–16 samples.

The immigrant sample had a total of 70 respondents: 31 interviewed during 2012–13 (21 Brazilians and 10 Dominicans), and 39 interviewed during 2015–16 (15 Brazilians, 14 Dominicans, and 10 Salvadorans). These are three of Boston's largest immigrant groups that have different migration histories to the United States and a range of documentation statuses. Dominicans have migrated to Boston since the 1960s and are typically LPRs or naturalized citizens. However, Salvadorans and Brazilians began migrating in the 1980s in response to political and economic crises in their home countries. Although some Salvadorans received TPS status, the majority of Salvadorans and Brazilians are undocumented. Dominicans, Brazilians, and Salvadorans also are from different parts of Latin America and are racialized as Latinos, which shapes their incorporation and health care experiences.[11] These interviews assessed: (1) the immigrant profile; (2) self-reported physical/mental health pre-migration and in the United States; and (3) insurance coverage/health care access pre-migration and in the United States. See table 2 for immigrant respondents' demographics.

To assess institutional factors that shape immigrants' health care experiences, thirty-eight health care professionals were interviewed at The Boston Health Coalition (BHC),[12] a system of safety net hospitals and clinics reputed for providing quality care to minority populations. The

10. As of 2012–13, Chapter 58 health reform had been implemented for six years.
11. Salvadorans were added in 2015–16 as some of them may have had TPS that entitled them to certain benefits from which Brazilian and Dominican noncitizens were excluded.
12. This is a pseudonym for the organization. Nineteen interviews each were conducted during 2012–13 and 2015–16.

Table 1   Respondent Sample Sizes (Total *N* = 153)

Stakeholder Group	Pre-ACA: 2012–2013	Post-ACA: 2015–2016
Immigrants	*N* = 31	*N* = 39
Brazilians	21	15
Dominicans	10	14
Salvadorans	N/A	10
Health Care Providers at BHC	*N* = 19	*N* = 19
Physicians	5	6
Medical interpreters	4	4
Other medical staff	10	9
Immigrant/Health Organizations	*N* = 20	*N* = 25
Brazilian	6	4
Dominican	2	4
Salvadoran	N/A	2
General immigrant organizations	3	5
Health organizations	9	7
City/state officials	0	3
Total	**70**	**83**

thirty-eight respondents were physicians, medical interpreters, social case workers, and psychiatrists across eight different BHC sites (see table 3). Interviews examined respondents' perceptions regarding: (1) difficulties serving immigrants; (2) availability of multilingual staff; (3) influence of health reforms—Chapter 58 and ACA—on serving patients; (4) health problems of immigrant patients; and (5) how being an immigrant affects their patients.

Lastly, to examine how immigration policy and local sociopolitical context influenced immigrants' health care access, interviews were conducted with forty-five employees of immigrant and health advocacy organizations that served different immigrant populations, or were health advocacy organizations that assisted Massachusetts residents in health insurance enrollment.[13] These interviews assessed: (1) sociopolitical climate for immigrants; (2) enforcement of state/federal immigration policy; and (3) difficulties that immigrants face living in Boston and accessing the health care system.

Study respondents were recruited through community events at immigrant and health advocacy organizations. Purposive snowball sampling

13. Twenty interviews were conducted in the 2012–13 period and twenty-five interviews during 2015–16.

Table 2 Immigrant Sample Demographics

Demographics	2012–2013 Immigrant Sample (N = 31)		2015–2016 Immigrant Sample (N = 39)		
	Brazilians (N = 21)	Dominicans (N = 10)	Brazilians (N = 15)	Dominicans (N = 14)	Salvadorans (N = 10)
Gender (# women)	12	5	8	10	6
Median age (years)	40	55	43	56	40
Average time in US (years)	12	14	10	21	19
Documentation Status					
- Current undocumented (N)	6	3	6	0	5
- Current visa/green card holders (N)	14	4	8	11	4
- Current naturalized citizens (N)	1	3	1	3	1
Health Insurance Coverage					
- Uninsured (N)	1	0	2	2	3
- Health safety net (N)	7	2	4	1	4
- Mass Health (N)	4	6	6	9	2
- Commonwealth Care (N)	1	0	0	0	1
- Private (N)	8	2	3	2	0

Table 3 BHC Respondent Demographics

Demographics	2012–2013 Sample (N = 19)	2015–2016 Sample (N = 19)
Gender (number of women)	14	14
Average age (years)	47	47
Number of years at BHC	13	13
Ethnoracial Classification		
- White (N)	9	10
- Black (N)	2	1
- Latino/Hispanic (N)	7	4
- Asian American (N)	0	1
- Other (N)	1	3

was especially effective amid community concerns regarding immigration enforcement and anti-immigrant sentiment during data collection. For the immigrant sample, women and men who had been in the United States for at least one year and were ages twenty-five to sixty were recruited, as these individuals were more likely to have adapted and to have used the health care system. The BHC respondents were medical professionals with mostly Brazilian, Dominican, Salvadoran, and/or other immigrant patients. Interviews were conducted in Brazilian Portuguese, Spanish, or English, typically lasting sixty minutes, and were audio-recorded and transcribed.[14]

For analysis, each interview transcript was imported into NVivo software, and an extensive list of codes was developed, with one- to three-word phrases describing how respondents felt documentation status influenced immigrants' health care experiences. Sub-codes were created that corresponded to each stakeholder group to compare perspectives across immigrants, health care professionals, and organization employees. Each transcript was re-read and all words, phrases, and sentences were organized under the associated codes, until all of the transcripts were analyzed. Each interview was analyzed in the language in which it was conducted to minimize the loss of nuances in translation. The findings presented reflect the perceptions of the stakeholder groups even if they may not directly correspond to eligibility for coverage based on health policy.

Access to the stakeholder groups allowed for qualitative exploration of the experiences of Brazilian, Dominican, and Salvadoran immigrants, who are underrepresented in immigration, health, and policy research. The data were collected in Boston, which is a progressive city that benefited from health reform prior to the ACA. However, previous studies of the Massachusetts health reform before ACA implementation in 2014 were used to project the potential national impact of the ACA. Although this small nonrandom sample limits the generalizability of the results, the findings may have implications for understanding how various populations navigate the health care system under health reform.

Findings

Results reveal that immigrants' awareness of their marginalized documentation status minimizes their enrollment in and use of health coverage even when they have eligibility. This awareness stems primarily from all stakeholders' perceptions that: (1) the intersection of different types of

---

14. Immigrants' interview anecdotes are translated from Brazilian Portuguese or Spanish.

public policy limits immigrants' health care access; (2) using local health care services may lead to deportation or jeopardize future federal legalization proceedings; and (3) increased local and federal immigration enforcement indirectly affects immigrants' health due to receiving delayed or no care. These concerns increase fear within immigrant communities that diminishes the effectiveness of inclusive local-level health reforms. Each of these concerns is discussed here, with interview anecdotes.

Regarding respondents' perceptions of how policy shapes immigrants' health care access, the different stakeholder groups often discussed how the intersection of policy—at municipal, state, and federal levels—as well as among health, immigration, and welfare policy, limited access to health care at the local level. Because these policies shift constantly, some stakeholders acknowledged that their perceptions of the impact of policies on immigrants may not always be accurate. Nevertheless, immigrants tend to err on the side of policies being punitive and alter their routines accordingly. This means that sometimes they will not use benefits despite being eligible for them. Regardless of whether policies were passed at the federal, state, or municipal levels, these policies are enacted and "lived" locally, affecting immigrants' immediate surroundings. Among respondents, the multifaceted intersection of policy was most apparent when it came to undocumented immigrants' inability to obtain driver's licenses under current state law, which limited their mobility. Federally, the 2005 Real ID Act was passed to standardize driver's licenses and government-issued identification (DHS 2015). Although states must verify "evidence of lawful status," they can issue licenses to undocumented immigrants. Only ten states currently do, and Massachusetts is not one (Pew Charitable Trusts 2015).

As Boston's public transportation system is not the most efficient, some immigrants feel they must drive without licenses to maintain their livelihoods, attend medical appointments, and transport family members to school, work, etc. This palpable risk leads to significant fear of law enforcement since being pulled over by police could lead to arrest and deportation. José, a Salvadoran immigrant, talked about the difficulty that driving illegally poses:

> If a person doesn't have [papers], is not legal, you cannot get a driver's license, you cannot have a Social Security number, or get loans if you need credit. These things, I think, make life more difficult.

This fear was more often expressed by Brazilian and Salvadoran immigrants who were more likely to be undocumented and consequently unable to obtain driver's licenses. As Dominican respondents were usually LPRs or naturalized citizens, the inability to legally drive did not affect them in the same way. Thus, each ethnic group's immigration history and related documentation status led to different experiences under Massachusetts driving policy.

Intersecting policies also complicate lawmakers' compliance with federal policy alongside competing goals to create access for federally ineligible immigrants. Immigrant advocacy organizations and Boston government officials have petitioned Massachusetts lawmakers to pass a Safe Driver Bill that would require every motorist to have a license regardless of documentation status. Respondents from advocacy organizations perceive that the current state administration has been unsupportive of the Safe Driver Bill or other proposed bills that would benefit immigrants. At the same time, the Boston mayor's office recently created an Office of Immigrant Advancement to make the city more welcoming to immigrants, illustrating how state and municipal legislators are on opposing sides of this issue. Darlene, a representative from the office, discussed the challenge of providing resources for Boston immigrants amid state and federal constraints:

> There are many offices that receive a significant amount of federal funding that are tied to federal policy. There is not much our office can do except give an opinion on it. If you're undocumented, it's very hard to get any amount of services that come through federal dollars. The policies are already set and we have to know what they are and be able to navigate people when they come. The state has a fairly new governor [and] the change in eligibility for Health Safety Net is something that was very significant. The governor does not support driver's license[s] for the undocumented. The mayor was a co-sponsor [as a previous state representative], but it's something that the mayor is where he is and the governor is where he is.

Being on conflicting sides affects policy making and implementation, which leaves potential beneficiaries hanging in the balance. And immigrants are especially vulnerable to being left out of the policy equation, although not necessarily intentionally so in Massachusetts.

Another concern that stakeholders mentioned as minimizing immigrants' health care access was immigrants' perceptions that their use of health care services would lead to deportation or jeopardize future legalization proceedings for themselves or relatives applying for LPR status or citizenship. This concern has been noted in previous research due to the 1996 PRWORA and IIRIRA reforms that represented a more restrictive intersection between the immigration, welfare, and health care systems

(Fox 2016; Park 2011). Concerns about this intersection, especially for Brazilian and Salvadoran noncitizens, created fear that using services and inability to pay for services could lead to deportation. This perception was also expressed among health care providers and immigrant/health advocacy organization employees. Maria, a Brazilian immigrant, told me how this affected her health care behaviors:

> Every time I would [consider going to the doctor,] I thought I would get like a $2,000 bill and if I did not pay, the police would go to my house and deport me. Like when you are illegal you are afraid. You do not know that Homeland Security is not attached to [health care system]. So I would be, really I was very afraid to have [medical] debt because you know immigration forces will find me and kick me out of the country.

Unaware that there was no direct connection between Immigration and Customs Enforcement (ICE) and the health care system, Maria believed she would be deported for inability to pay medical bills. She revealed later in the interview that, instead of receiving treatment in a formal health care setting, she had a friend in Brazil send her medication.

Elisa, a Dominican immigrant, also made a connection between immigrants' use of health services and deportation, although she does not feel personally affected by this as a long-term LPR:

> Those who don't have papers experience a lot of discrimination, especially when you have children because you cannot go see a doctor or have insurance. Sometimes, your child gets sick and you have to take the risk of getting him to the doctor without knowing if you will be deported to your country.

The implicit and underlying theme in Elisa and Maria's quotes as well as the first finding regarding the intersection of public policy allude to the health implications for immigrants. The impact of policy and misconceptions about the relationship between deportation and health service use is that local immigrants seek delayed health care or none at all. Respondents across all groups also mentioned how heightened racialized immigration enforcement and anti-immigrant sentiment at the national level is affecting local immigrants' health through shaping their health care behaviors.[15] Compared to the interviews conducted during 2012–13,

---

15. The Obama administration's enforcement of existing immigration policy alongside increased racialized profiling by law and immigration enforcement yielded a record number of deportations for Latino and black male immigrants (Golash-Boza 2015). Deportations may increase under the Trump administration given his campaign promises to get tough on immigration.

stakeholders interviewed in 2015–16 felt that the social climate for immigrants was comparatively worse, specifically citing the ethnoracial profiling of immigrants. A Salvadoran immigrant was shot and killed by police in April 2016 while a legal Mexican immigrant (presumed to be undocumented) was attacked by two young white men in August 2015 (Anderson and Sacchetti 2016; Walker 2015).

Whenever ICE raids occur in immigrant communities, or immigrants hear through social media that ICE will be patrolling certain areas, immigrants do not leave home for work or anywhere else. Terrorism concerns also yield fear for immigrants when they see police officers checking passengers in subway stations even though local law enforcement has no immigration enforcement authority. Whatever the circumstance may be, multiple respondents in each group discussed how this decreases the likelihood that immigrants will seek health care. Meghan, a social case worker at the Boston Health Coalition, shared:

> We face issues with patients who are facing deportation because they were coming to the clinic and they were pulled over. [When] the new law [Secure Communities] was put in place that the police were going and stopping people and doing raids and stuff. So a lot of our patients got caught. We had a patient who was coming to the clinic one day, and they called to say, "I'm not going to make it to the visit because on my way to the clinic I saw a police car, so I'm turning around." So they just turned around. So all that plays in with the patients.[16]

While BHC providers like Meghan and immigrant respondents who are BHC patients consider BHC sites to be culturally competent, safe spaces to receive care, immigrants' concerns about arriving at BHC without being apprehended by police sometimes outweigh their medical needs. This has also been the case in other parts of the country where immigrants are afraid to receive care at culturally competent FQHCs due to immigration enforcement (Hacker et al. 2012; López-Sanders 2013; Marrow 2012).

Given that immigrants are excluded from ACA provisions and consequently more likely to be uninsured, the remaining health care option available to most is emergency departments (ED) (Newton et al. 2008; Tarraf, Vega, and González 2014). But, immigrants' ED use is lower than

16. Secure Communities (S-Comm) allows information-sharing between local authorities and Immigration and Customs Enforcement (ICE) when immigrants are arrested. S-Comm sends the fingerprints of locally arrested individuals to the Federal Bureau of Investigation (FBI) and ICE for placement in a database. If the arrested individual is an undocumented immigrant, ICE may ask the local authorities to detain the individual, after which s/he may be deported. S-Comm has created fear in immigrant communities (Golash-Boza 2015; Hacker et al. 2012).

that of naturalized and native-born citizens (Tarraf, Vega, and González 2014). Among most BHC health care professionals and a few immigrants in this study, ED use is not considered to be "safer" in terms of immigration enforcement, as patients may still be stopped on their way to culturally competent EDs like those at BHC. But, some immigrant respondents considered ED use to be cheaper, especially for low-income patients, who, despite having low/no co-pays, are unable to afford them for physician visits and prescription medications. Meghan, the BHC employee quoted earlier, also provided specific examples of how low-income immigrant patients came to BHC EDs to avoid the co-pays associated with a visit to their physicians. Despite having publicly subsidized coverage, immigrants in this study were unaware that their ED use would result in higher health care costs for the state and health care facilities, who paid for those ED services. Thus, affordability was another motivating factor (alongside immigration enforcement concerns) in ED use compared to other types of health services among immigrants in this study.

Alcione, an employee at a community organization that assists Brazilian immigrants with social services enrollment, also spoke about how immigration enforcement fears causes her constituents to put their health at risk by not seeking care, except under dire circumstances:

> I saw a post [Facebook] that said "I live in Rhode Island, please don't drive on I-495 at night if you don't have a license. ICE is pulling over everyone." [This post is] causing a new terror in our communities. And what about health? If a person can't drive on I-495, and is this afraid, they will not go to the doctor if they live in Marlborough [MA] and have to go to Worcester [MA]. But the police have nothing to do with health care, and people don't know that.[17]

Despite living in Massachusetts and being eligible for health coverage, some immigrants will not use health services due to fear generated by federal immigration policy and assumptions they will be profiled and deported en route to receiving care.

Discussion and Health Equity Implications

Boston and Massachusetts have reputations for being progressive and more immigrant-inclusive relative to other parts of the country. But, they are not immune to the broader national sociopolitical climate that has become

17. Rhode Island borders Massachusetts and many people there cross the state lines every day.

increasingly anti-immigrant and is affected by budget constraints. These national trends are shaping local immigrants' ability to apply for health coverage and use health services. Concerns among immigrants, health care providers, and immigrant/health organization employees in this study suggest that immigrants, particularly the undocumented, are delaying or not seeking health care despite their local-level eligibility. The qualitative examination of the region between 2012 and 2013 and 2015 and 2016 presented here is one of the first to demonstrate how macro-level changes in health reform and anti-immigrant attitudes is affecting local immigrants at the micro level.

The findings also reveal the indelible relationship between local, state, and federal policies, and their impact on immigrants' health care in Boston. This intersection of policy creates a perfect storm of systematic de jure and informal de facto exclusion for immigrants, many of whom are low-income and ethnoracial minorities. This nuanced combination of de jure and de facto discrimination has severe health equity implications for immigrants not only in Massachusetts, but also across the country where most immigrants are excluded from health coverage and live in overtly anti-immigrant states.

Under the ACA and other federal policies that limit noncitizens' access to public benefits, immigrants' exclusion represents legally sanctioned discrimination on the basis of documentation status. Given that the historic de jure race-based discrimination of the pre–Civil Rights era has influenced contemporary health disparities for ethnoracial minorities, similar legal discrimination toward immigrants will likely have a profound impact on their health care access and outcomes for years to come. Although Massachusetts immigrants fare better than immigrants elsewhere through their legal inclusion (for the time being) in the state's health policy, their federal legal exclusion in other types of policy reduces their ability to fully benefit from their health care inclusion.

Legal distinctions between classes of individuals based on documentation status also spills over into the social realm, affecting interpersonal relations and facilitating de facto discrimination in people's health care experiences. This was the case for some immigrants in the study, who felt the weight of being mistreated by "Americans" due to their presumed immigrant status. Implicit in this mistreatment was a sense of "otherness" that stemmed from being perceived and racialized as a foreigner, which might have led to being profiled en route to receiving health services. Given that Brazilians, Dominicans, and Salvadorans are racialized differently on the basis of their phenotypes, each group's perceptions of their "otherness" is tied to their ability to physically blend into the white population. Though Brazilians in the sample had physical features that spanned from white to black, lighter Brazilians' ability to pass for white made them less likely to be profiled than darker Brazilians and Dominicans, who are racialized as black, and Salvadorans, who are racialized as Latino.[18] The privilege of white Americans alongside the social stigma of blacks and Latinos differentially affects Brazilian, Dominican, and Salvadoran immigrants' encounters with law and immigration enforcement, health care professionals, and everyday Americans.

The heterogeneity of the Latino immigrant sample also provides insight into how language differences may be implicit barriers to care that have not been explored in depth in other studies. The fact that Brazilians speak Portuguese and some Salvadorans speak indigenous languages means that enrollment forms and interpreter assistance available only in English or Spanish further minimize their ability to access coverage and care. Thus, lawmakers and health care providers should also be careful to consider how the diversity of more recent immigrants creates linguistic and cultural needs that are different from immigrant groups with a larger presence and established history in the country.

Additionally, when considering that most contemporary immigrants are people of color, the ongoing significance of race and ethnicity in US society makes them more likely to experience de facto racial discrimination (Golash-Boza 2015). These study findings illustrate how distinctions encoded in policy also create social, symbolic, and racialized boundaries between eligible citizens and ineligible noncitizens (Marrow and Joseph 2015). And as health disparities in the post–Civil Rights era suggest that de facto racial discrimination continues to drive those disparities, it is likely the same will occur for immigrant-based de facto discrimination.

Aside from highlighting the nuances of de jure and de facto discrimination, the findings also reveal the challenges associated with maintaining an inclusive local health reform for a population whose access to benefits has been federally curtailed since the 1980s. A consequence of Massachusetts' commitment to providing public coverage to its income-eligible residents of any documentation status is that the state's health care costs are the nation's highest (Song and Landon 2012). This has led lawmakers to make difficult decisions to meet the state's fiscal responsibilities each budget year (Song and Landon 2012). Historically, those decisions have

18. Racial inequality in Brazil has granted white Brazilians more structural access for immigration compared to brown and black Brazilians (Joseph 2015).

come at the expense of federally ineligible immigrants and low-income state residents (Joseph 2016). Over the years, the income eligibility bar for public coverage has been reduced, making federally ineligible immigrants more vulnerable to losing coverage through programs like the Health Safety Net.

While respondents have noticed a shift to less inclusive state-level policies that they fear will affect immigrant, ethnoracial, and low-income communities, they all expressed a perception that Massachusetts is in a much better position on these issues than other states. This sentiment was echoed often when stakeholders in each group provided anecdotal stories of immigrants who considered moving to other states and learned they would be unable to access the same types of benefits. Respondents also reflected on how being in a progressive state and having a strong coalition among various nonprofit organizations translates to greater receptiveness and communication from state policy makers on a range of issues.

The Massachusetts case also illustrates the health equity implications for other marginalized groups nationwide when considering the impact of imperfect ACA implementation. This is particularly the case for low-income and/or ethnoracial minority populations. Just as documentation status and income delineate health coverage options in Massachusetts, these factors worked similarly in the national-level ACA. A key difference was that eligible citizens' exclusion in non-Medicaid expansion states could have been overcome within the framework of the ACA. But, with conservative lawmakers' promises to repeal the ACA, eligible citizens' exclusion may spread to Medicaid expansion states. But, most immigrants, who were overtly excluded from the original law, will remain excluded (Marrow and Joseph 2015). In both cases, eligible citizens in non-expansion states and most immigrants in all states will be excluded on a de jure basis. However, the stakes of exclusion for citizens will not be as high as for immigrants, as citizens can currently access other benefits (e.g., welfare) that immigrants cannot. Citizens also will not be subject to deportation for being public charges when using benefits or accruing high health care costs.

Just as race influences the experiences of contemporary immigrants accessing health care, gender and age also play a role. Some populations are considered more vulnerable, like women and children, which entitles them to certain federal health care benefits regardless of documentation status. Income-eligible children can receive coverage through the Children's Health Insurance Program while pregnant immigrant women can receive emergency Medicaid for prenatal care and delivery. However, men who are undocumented or in other federally ineligible categories cannot receive similar benefits. These dynamics of documentation status, income, race/ethnicity, and gender are reflected within the context of Boston under inclusive state and federal health reforms. But these factors, in addition to state of residence, also shape eligibility and delineate health coverage among the national population. Consequently, these factors exacerbated health disparities under the ACA (Garfield and Damico 2016). Without the ACA, these disparities will worsen.

Finally, Boston (and Massachusetts) may be considered a best-case scenario for continuing to provide state-funded coverage for federally ineligible immigrants amid budget constraints. Massachusetts is not alone in this regard, as other countries have made efforts to include certain, usually documented, immigrants in their national coverage provisions (Gray and van Ginneken 2012). The situation for undocumented immigrants is more precarious, although the United States has the largest undocumented population among Western nations (Gray and van Ginneken 2012). Canada's universal health coverage program includes documented immigrants, who fare similarly to Canadian citizens and insured American citizens in terms of health care access (Siddiqi, Zuberi, and Nguyen 2009). But, undocumented immigrants are ineligible for national health insurance (Elgersma 2008). Unauthorized immigrants have access to emergency care in 20 of 27 European Union countries as of 2011 (Björngren-Cuadra and Cattacin 2011). However, they must pay for this emergency care in 11 of these 20 countries (Björngren-Cuadra and Cattacin 2011). Beyond emergency care, there is considerable variation in what individual countries provide for immigrants in their jurisdictions (Björngren-Cuadra and Cattacin 2011; Gray and van Ginneken 2012). Much of this care, as in the United States, is delineated by certain conditions, such as having been previously documented (Gray and van Ginneken 2012).

Like Massachusetts, EU countries struggle to fund health coverage for federally ineligible immigrants. Budget downturns usually yield cuts to such coverage, illustrating the expendability of this population. Even when coverage is provided, immigrant populations in these places still face challenges navigating the system and finding culturally competent and linguistically compatible care (i.e., interpreters) (Long, Goin, and Lynch 2013; PICUM 2011). While access to coverage is essential for producing health equity, simplifying enrollment procedures, making related correspondence and assistance available in multiple languages, and having multilingual and ethnically diverse health care professionals also make the health care system more accessible. But, given that immigrants tend to arrive in the United States with better health and then face prolonged periods of non-access to care, which leads to more expensive emergency room and treatment costs as they age, policies that provide accessible care now will save money in the future. They also will generate health equity for a significant global demographic.

Immigrants' current underinsurance (in Massachusetts) and exclusion from the ACA on the basis of documentation status illustrates how this sociopolitical construction (alongside race, ethnicity, and income) facilitates de jure as well as de facto discrimination for this group. This article has illustrated how the intersection of multiple policy domains increases social inequality in health care access in Boston and reflects a similar citizen-noncitizen divide in American society. The Boston case offers insights for other locales that aim to incorporate inclusive reforms despite the ACA's exclusions for most immigrants. The inclusive Boston case also allows researchers, policy makers, and the general population to imagine the starkly greater vulnerability that immigrants, particularly those of color, around the nation may experience when they are overtly excluded from state- and federal-level reforms.

Consequently, President Donald Trump and conservative federal lawmakers' promises to repeal the ACA have generated concerns about how such action will affect ACA beneficiaries and the larger health care system. Repealing the ACA will likely undo any health equity gains made in expansion and non-expansion states, as some aspects of the law (e.g., preexisting conditions, young adult coverage through age 26) benefited people around the country. Furthermore, 20 million people who currently receive coverage through the Medicaid expansion or health exchanges may lose their insurance, especially if conservative federal lawmakers do not develop a replacement plan before repealing (Blumenthal and Collins 2016).

Even without the ACA, President Trump's overtly anti-immigrant policies will likely result in fewer federally eligible immigrants using health or other social services, particularly as immigration enforcement and deportations are anticipated to increase under his administration (Chozick 2017). Amid such policy changes, the social and symbolic boundaries around immigrants will be brightened, increasing their vulnerability and exclusion. As for Massachusetts, repealing the ACA may mean reverting to the state's 2006 reform. However, the state would have to generate additional revenue to compensate for the budget shortfall from federal Medicaid expansion funds. State lawmakers will likely remain committed to maintaining "universal" coverage, but will make difficult budget decisions regarding who to provide coverage for and how much to provide. If history is any indicator, federally ineligible (and perhaps some eligible) immigrants and low-income residents may be expendable to maintain coverage for (middle-income) citizen residents. Thus, the health equity implications for Massachusetts may be less severe than for the nation, but disparities in coverage and care will likely increase among the state and country's most vulnerable populations if a suitable ACA replacement policy is not passed and implemented.

▪ ▪ ▪

Tiffany D. Joseph is assistant professor of sociology and affiliated faculty in the Latin American and Caribbean Studies Center at Stony Brook University. Her research interests include: race, ethnicity, and migration in the Americas; the influence of immigration on the social construction of race in the United States; immigrants' health and health care access; immigration and health policy; and the experiences of minority faculty in academia. She is the author of *Race on the Move: Brazilian Migrants and the Global Reconstruction of Race* (Stanford University Press, 2015), and a member of the Scholars Strategy Network.
tiffany.joseph@stonybrook.edu

Acknowledgments

The author would like to thank the study participants as well as guest editors, fellow authors of this volume, and attendees of the 2016 Robert Wood Johnson Foundation Health Investigator Awards meeting for their constructive feedback on earlier versions of the manuscript.

References

Anderson, Travis, and Maria Sacchetti. 2016. "Everett Immigrant Fatally Shot by Police Is Mourned at Vigil." *Boston Globe*, April 26.

Batalova, Jeanne, Sarah Hooker, Randy Capps, James D. Bachmeier, and Erin Cox. 2013. "Deferred Action for Childhood Arrivals at the One-Year Mark." August. *Issue Brief* 8. Washington, DC: Migration Policy Institute.

Betancourt, James, and Matthew Bondaryk. 2014. "Addressing Disparities and Achieving Equity: Cultural Competence, Ethics, and Health-care Transformation." *Chest* 145, no. 1: 143–48.

Björngren-Cuadra, Carin, and Sandro Cattacin. 2011. "Policies on Health Care for Undocumented Migrants in the EU27 and Switzerland: Towards a Comparative Framework." Summary Report. Malmö, Sweden: Health Care in Nowhereland, Malmö University.

Blumenthal, David, and Sara Collins. 2016. "The Affordable Care Act in 2017: Challenges for President-Elect Trump and Congress." Commonwealth Fund Blog. Nov 10. www.commonwealthfund.org/publications/blog/2016/nov/challenges-for -president-elect-trump-and-congress.

Capps, Randy, and Michael Fix. 2013. "Immigration Reform: A Long Road to Citizenship and Insurance Coverage." *Health Affairs* 32, no. 4: 639–42.

Castañeda, Heide, and Milena A. Melo. 2014. "Health Care Access for Latino Mixed-Status Families: Barriers, Strategies, and Implications for Reform." *American Behavioral Scientist* 58, no. 14: 1891–1909.

Cheney, Kyle. 2014. "Mass. Ditches RomneyCare Exchange." *Politico.com*, May 5. www.politico.com/story/2014/05/massachusetts-romneycare-health-care-exchange -106362.

Chin, Michael, Deborah Gurewich, Kathy Muhr, Heather Posner, Jennifer Rosinski, Elise LaFlamme, and Audrey Gasteier. 2016. "The Remaining Uninsured in Massachusetts: Experiences of Individuals Living without Health Insurance Coverage." Boston: Blue Cross Blue Shield of Massachusetts Foundation.

Chozick, Amy. 2017. "Raids of Illegal Immigrants Bring Harsh Memories, and Strong Fears." *New York Times*, January 2.

Decker, Sandra L. 2012. "In 2011 Nearly One-Third of Physicians Said They Would Not Accept New Medicaid Patients, but Rising Fees May Help." *Health Affairs* 31, no. 8: 1673–79.

DHS (US Department of Homeland Security). 2015. "REAL ID Enforcement in Brief." Washington, DC: Department of Homeland Security.

Donelson, Katelynn. 2015. "Medical Repatriation: The Dangerous Intersection of Health Care Law and Immigration." *Health Care Law and Policy* 347: 18J.

Elgersma, Sandra. 2008. "Immigration Status and Legal Entitlement to Insured Health Services." October 28. Parliament of Canada, Political and Social Affairs Division.

Evans, Marissa. 2016. "California Opens Door to Health Insurance for Undocumented Immigrants." Commonwealth Fund, June 27. New York: Commonwealth Fund.

Fox, Cybelle. 2016. "Unauthorized Welfare: The Origins of Immigrant Status Restrictions in American Social Policy." *Journal of American History* 102, no. 4: 1051–74.

Garfield, Rachel, and Anthony Damico. 2016. "The Coverage Gap: Uninsured Poor Adults in States That Do Not Expand Medicaid—An Update." Menlo Park, CA: Kaiser Family Foundation.

Golash-Boza, Tanya. 2015. *Deported: Immigrant Policing, Disposable Labor and Global Capitalism*. New York: New York University Press.

Gray, Bradford H., and Ewout van Ginneken. 2012. "Health Care for Undocumented Migrants: European Approaches." Issues in International Health Policy. Commonwealth Fund pub. 1650, Vol. 33. New York: Commonwealth Fund.

Hacker, Karen, Jocelyn Chu, Lisa Arsenault, and Robert P. Marlin. 2012. "Provider's Perspectives on the Impact of Immigration and Customs Enforcement (ICE) Activity on Immigrant Health." *Journal of Health Care for the Poor and Underserved* 23: 651–65.

HHS (US Department of Health and Human Services). 2015. "Sex, Race, and Ethnic Diversity of U.S. Health Occupations (2010–2012)." Washington, DC: Health Services and Resources Administration.

IIRIRA Illegal Immigration Reform and Immigrant Responsibility Act. 1996. Public Law 104–208, 104th Cong. 1st sess. (September 30, 1996).

IOM (Institute of Medicine). 2002. "Unequal Treatment: Confronting Racial and Ethnic Disparities in Health Care." Washington, DC: Institute of Medicine.

Joseph, Tiffany D. 2015. *Race on the Move: Brazilian Migrants and the Global Reconstruction of Race*. Palo Alto: Stanford University Press.

Joseph, Tiffany D. 2016. "What Healthcare Reform Means for Immigrants: A Comparison of the Affordable Care Act and Massachusetts Health Reforms." *Journal of Health Politics, Policy and Law* 41, no. 1: 101–16.

Long, Sharon, Dana Goin, and Victoria Lynch. 2013. "Reaching the Remaining Uninsured in Massachusetts: Challenges and Opportunities." Boston: Blue Cross Blue Shield of Massachusetts Foundation.

López-Sanders, Laura. 2013. "Unintended Penalties: How Brokered Access Influences Health Care Services for Undocumented Latino Immigrants." Paper presented at the annual meeting of the Robert Wood Johnson Foundation Health Policy Scholars Program, Princeton, NJ, June 6.

Marrow, Helen B. 2012. "Deserving to a Point: Unauthorized Immigrants in San Francisco's Universal Access Healthcare Model." *Social Science and Medicine* 74: 846–54.

Marrow, Helen, and Tiffany D. Joseph. 2015. "Excluded and Frozen Out: Unauthorized Immigrants' (Non) Access to Care after Health Care Reforms." *Journal of Ethnic and Migration Studies* 41, no. 14: 2253–73.

Mass.gov. 2016. "Announcement about Health Safety Net Changes." April 6. www.masshealthmtf.org/news/announcement-about-health-safety-net-changes.

Mass Legal Services. 2016. "Blowing a Hole in the Health Safety Net: EOHHS Notice of Proposed Rules." www.masslegalservices.org/content/health-safety-net-cuts-public-hearing-feb-26-2016.

McDonough, John. 2016. "Behind the Massachusetts Health Connector's Rehab." *Commonwealth Magazine*, April 6 https://commonwealthmagazine.org/health-care/behind-the-massachusetts-health-connectors-rehab/.

Newton, Manya F., Carla C. Keirns, Rebecca Cunningham, Rodney A. Hayward, and Rachel Stanley. 2008. "Uninsured Adults Presenting to US Emergency Departments: Assumptions vs Data." *Journal of the American Medical Association* 300, no. 16: 1914–24.

NYLPI (New York Lawyers for the Public Interest). 2012. "Discharge, Deportation, and Dangerous Journeys: A Study on the Practice of Medical Repatriation." Center for Social Justice and Health Justice Program, December. Fairfield, CT: Seton Hall

University Law School. https://law.shu.edu/ProgramsCenters/PublicIntGovServ /CSJ/upload/final-med-repat-report-2012.pdf.

Park, Lisa Sun-Hee. 2011. *Entitled to Nothing: The Struggle for Immigrant Health Care in the Age of Welfare Reform.* New York: New York University Press.

Patel, Kavita, and John McDonough. 2010. "From Massachusetts to 1600 Pennsyl-vania Avenue: Aboard the Health Reform Express." *Health Affairs* 29, no. 6: 1106–11.

Pew Charitable Trusts. 2015. "Deciding Who Drives: State Choices surrounding Unauthorized Immigrants and Driver's Licenses." Washington, DC: Pew Research.

PICUM (Platform for International Cooperation on Undocumented Migrants). 2011. "Undocumented Migrants' Health Needs and Strategies to Access Health Care in 17 EU Countries and Switzerland." Summary Report, 2nd ed. Workpackage No. 6. files.nowhereland.info/756.pdf.

Portes, Alejandro, Patricia Fernández-Kelly, and Donald W. Light. 2012. "Life on the Edge: Immigrants Confront the American Health System." *Ethnic and Racial Studies* 35, no. 1: 3–22.

Schumann, John. 2016. "When the Cost of Care Triggers a Medical Deportation." April 9. Washington, DC: NPR.

Sentell, Tetine, and Kathryn Braun. 2012."Low Health Literacy, Limited English Proficiency, and Health Status in Asians, Latinos, and Other Racial/Ethnic Groups in California." *Journal of Health Communication: International Perspectives* 17: 82–99.

Shavers, Vickie, Fagan Pebbles, Dionne Jones, William M. P. Klein, Josephine Boy-ington, Carmen Moten, and Edward Rorie. 2012. "The State of Research on Racial/ Ethnic Discrimination in the Receipt of Health Care." *American Journal of Public Health* 102, no. 5: 953–66.

Siddiqi, Arjumand, Daniyal Zuberi, and Quynh Nguyen. 2009. "The Role of Health Insurance for Explaining Immigrant versus Non-Immigrant Disparities in Access to Health Care: Comparing the United States to Canada." *Social Science and Medi-cine* 69, no. 10: 1452–59.

Song, Zirui, and Bruce Landon. 2012. "Controlling Health Care Spending: The Massachusetts Experiment." *New England Journal of Medicine* 366, no.17: 1560–61.

Tarraf, Wassim, William Vega, and Hector M. González. 2014. "Emergency Depart-ment Services Use among Immigrant and Non-Immigrant Groups in the United States." *Journal of Immigrant and Minority Health* 16: 595–606.

Walker, Adrian. 2015. "'Passionate' Trump Fans behind Homeless Man's Beating?" *Boston Globe*, August 21.

Warner, David C. 2012. "Access to Health Care Services for Immigrants in the USA: From the Great Society to the 2010 Health Reform Act and After." *Ethnic and Racial Studies* 35, no.1: 40–55.

Ybarra, Vickie D., Lisa M. Sanchez, and Gabriel R. Sanchez. 2015. "Anti-Immigrant Anxieties in State Policy: The Great Recession and Punitive Immigration Policy in the American States, 2005–2012." *State Politics and Policy Quarterly.* doi: 10.1177/1532440015605815.

Zoellner, Emily R. 2010. "Medical Repatriation: Examining the Legal and Ethical Implications of an Emerging Practice." *Washington University Journal of Law and Policy* 32: 515.

How the ACA Addressed Health Equity and What Repeal Would Mean

Colleen M. Grogan
University of Chicago

Abstract This commentary reviews the many different ways the Affordable Care Act (ACA) explicitly and implicitly attempted to improve health equity, and then assesses how the Republican proposal to repeal and replace the ACA (the proposed American Health Care Act) would impact efforts to improve health equity. Although the American health care system still had a long way to go to achieve health equity, it may be argued that the ACA was a major step forward in creating new programs and regulations that had the potential to improve health equity. In stark contrast, Trumpcare makes no mention of health equity as a goal and—if passed—would result in an increase in health inequity. It would shamefully represent the first time in modern US history that a major federal health reform bill would actually move us further away from creating more equal access to health care coverage and toward reduced health equity.

Keywords Trumpcare, ACA, health inequity

In a bill that is 906 pages long one might think that the Affordable Care Act (ACA) would impact many different facets of our health care system, and of course it does, despite the media and political focus on the coverage components of the bill. While the coverage components are crucially important for improving health equity in the United States, the ACA provided new provisions across the policy spectrum to address health equity in a multipronged approach.

As discussed in the Introduction of this special issue, there are multiple ways to approach achieving health equity: from focusing on creating a more inclusive and fair decision-making process to improve health equity to focusing on direct investments in vulnerable communities to create a

Journal of Health Politics, Policy and Law, Vol. 42, No. 5, October 2017
DOI 10.1215/03616878-3940508 © 2017 by Duke University Press

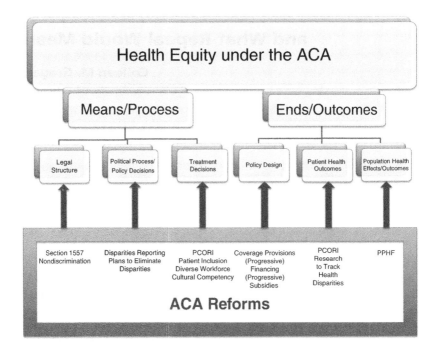

Figure 1 Health Equity under the ACA

more equal distribution of health outcomes. What should be fully appreciated about the ACA is that it indeed included provisions for improving health equity through creation of a fairer process and a more equal distribution of health outcomes, and also invested across multiple levels within the health care system (see fig. 1). In this short commentary I walk through some of the most important provisions of the law. This illustrates the magnitude of the ACA's intent to impact health equity. While we can debate how well various provisions would have improved health equity (or will improve equity in the absence of repeal), it is clear that improving health equity was (and continues to be) a central goal of the ACA, and a number of provisions were implemented to achieve that goal.

This is crucially important because you cannot begin to achieve a goal unless you place that goal in legislation, and create concrete implementation plans to begin the hard work. The ACA did that. Therefore, when the Congress debates total ACA repeal with or followed by a replacement bill (as is happening as this issue goes to press), it is important to grasp all that will be thrown out and how unlikely it is that health equity will be stated as a central goal of replacement legislation—much less the inclusion of provisions to achieve the goal.

How the ACA Addressed Health Equity

All ten titles of the Affordable Care Act contain some aspect concerning health equity.[1] There are thirty-five explicit mentions of "health disparities" in the Act—all specifying a particular effort to reduce or eliminate health disparities. Title I focuses primarily on reforms to the individual and group health insurance markets. There are numerous sections of Title I that deal explicitly with prohibiting various forms of discrimination.[2] As Rosenbaum and Schmucker discuss in this issue, Section 1557 (ACA § 1557[a]) is particularly important because it prohibits health insurers and health care providers not only from intentional discrimination, but also from engaging in unintentional behaviors that result in a disproportionate impact by race, ethnicity, gender, disability, or age (see also Watson 2012).

Title II deals primarily with specifications for improving access to the Medicaid program—what is now known as the Medicaid expansion. However, also included in this title is Section 2951, which details goals to improve maternal, infant, and early childhood home visiting programs for at-risk communities. This section not only requires states to submit a needs assessment to identify communities at risk, but also a plan for addressing these needs, which would "improve health care practices, *eliminate health disparities*, and improve health care system quality, efficiencies, and reduce costs" (p. 340, emphasis added).

Title III specifies a set of programs and principles for improving the quality and efficiency of health care where the goal of attempting to achieve health equity is clearly specified. Under directives to the Secretary of the Department of Health and Human Services (HHS) to develop a "National Strategy," one of the seven requirements listed states that "the Secretary shall ensure that priorities identified [will] . . . reduce health disparities across health disparity populations and geographic areas" (p. 378). Similar language is added for determining performance bonus payments for Medicare advantage plans, that is, that performance indicators would take into account reductions in health disparities (p. 448).

Particularly significant is the creation of the Prevention and Public Health Fund (PPHF) detailed under Title IV to "provide expanded and sustained national investments in prevention and public health, to improve

1. Title VIII, the CLASS Act, was officially repealed on January 1, 2013, so I will not discuss that title.

2. Section 2716, Prohibition of discrimination based on salary; Section 2704, Prohibition of preexisting condition exclusions or other discrimination based on health status; and Section 1557, Nondiscrimination.

health outcomes, and to enhance health care quality" (APHA 2017). Although the PPHF never received the full funding initially specified under the ACA in 2010, the establishment of this fund is significant in representing the first mandatory funding stream for public health from the federal government (Pollack 2011). Many studies attempting to pinpoint how best to improve health outcomes and reduce disparities point to investments in population health as key. Thus, it is noteworthy that a core part of PPHF's funding has gone to bolster the country's public health infrastructure—to create the basic components of a healthy community—as well as to prevent the spread of infectious diseases and control their outbreaks. In addition, PPHF dollars have gone directly to support "programs at the local, state, and federal levels that fight obesity, curb tobacco use, and increase access to preventive care services" (APHA 2017).

Title IV also created community transformation grants administered by the CDC, with the expressed purpose of creating healthy communities that would prioritize "strategies to reduce racial and ethnic disparities, including social, economic, and geographic determinants of health" (pp. 564–65). In the first year alone (2011), the CDC provided sixty-seven grants across thirty-six states. Most grants funded private-public partnerships across multiple sectors including schools, transportation, private businesses, and faith-based and nonprofit community-based organizations (CDC 2017).

Title V of the ACA is devoted to improving the health care workforce with specific attention to improving cultural competency and public health proficiency training to reduce health disparities (p. 628). The Patient-Centered Outcomes Research Institute (PCORI) was established under Title VI of the ACA. Its purpose has been to assist patients, providers, purchasers, and policy makers in making informed health decisions by advancing the quality of evidence of comparative clinical effectiveness information through rigorous research. The ACA specified gaps in knowledge regarding health disparities as an important indicator to be used when identifying research priorities (p. 729). Title VII—improving access to innovative medical therapies—contains three sections devoted to improving access to affordable medicines for children and underserved communities. And, finally, Section 10334 is devoted to issues pertaining to "Minority Health" under Title X.

These provisions, while glossed over here for the sake of brevity, when taken together, convey the breadth of attention given to improving health equity under the ACA (see fig. 1).[3] And yet, although these provisions are

---

3. Note these are not even all the provisions that address health equity in the ACA. For a discussion of other provisions not discussed here, see Fiscella (2011).

the least recognized related to the ACA and therefore worth highlighting here, I would be remiss in not mentioning the enormous progress the coverage components have made toward improving health equity. Providing coverage through the Medicaid expansion and health exchanges not only has created more equal access to health care services, but also has significantly redistributed the burden of health care costs. In particular, the ACA coverage expansions moved the US distribution of premium costs from extremely regressive (where the poor pay a higher proportion of their income for premiums compared to higher-income Americans) to a much more progressive distribution. This is especially true in the expansion states where premium burdens—the amount that individuals are expected to pay—were made logically progressive starting at zero and gradually increasing at each higher income level (Grogan 2015).

On the revenue side as well, the ACA has made the tax system more progressive. Individuals at the very high end of the income distribution (2 percent of taxpayers) were required to pay higher federal taxes, higher Medicare payroll taxes (by 0.9 percent), and increased taxes on unearned income (largely investments) by 3.8 percent (Rice 2011: 492). These new taxes—all imposed on the very wealthy relative to the remaining 98 percent of Americans—covered a significant portion (about 17 percent) of total funding needed to pay for expansions contained in the ACA (Dorn, Garrett, and Holahan 2014).

Finally, the ACA also includes progressively rated cost-sharing subsidies for people who earn up to 250 percent of the poverty line in the health care marketplaces (from 6 percent to 27 percent cost-sharing levels) (Health Policy Brief 2013). And, the ACA sets limits on the total out-of-pocket costs for marketplace plans ($6,600 for an individual plan and $13,200 for a family plan in 2015). The financing of these coverage provisions significantly lowered the financial burden of health care costs for low-income Americans, while at the same time creating more equitable access to health care services.

While the ACA had a long way to go to eliminate health disparities, it is important to take stock of all that was put in place to help improve health equity, especially in light of current proposals in Congress to repeal and replace the ACA. If the chief bill now before Congress—the so-called American Health Care Act that passed the House (which is all that has passed as of this writing in February 2017)—is passed, what would be lost, and would any gains toward health equity be achieved?

What Repeal and Replace Would Mean

Not surprisingly, repealing and replacing the ACA coverage provisions are the key foci of the reform proposal. The individual mandate, along with health care marketplaces and the subsidies for low-income individuals, would be repealed in favor of people purchasing health insurance *voluntarily* in the individual insurance market with the help of tax credits. While the Medicaid expansion would be an option for states to continue expanding coverage until the end of 2019, it also would then be repealed. At that point, Medicaid financing would be changed from a matching rate formula in which the federal government matches (50–82 percent of) the amounts that states contribute to the program to a per capita cap (PCC) in which the federal government provides a flat amount per person based on 2016 per-person expenditures. The bottom line is that switching to a PCC financing scheme will lower the amount of federal funding to the states for covering Medicaid expenses. The Center on Budget and Policy Priorities estimates that states would have to cover an additional $370 billion in Medicaid costs over the next ten years (Park, Aron-Dine, and Broaddus 2017). Finally, the taxation policies imposed on wealthy Americans to finance the ACA expansions would all be repealed with no tax policy replacements. The Joint Committee on Taxation estimates that repealing the ACA's tax directives will cost nearly $600 billion through 2026, and almost all of these savings would go to the very rich (Committee for a Responsible Federal Budget 2017; Mermin 2017) (see fig. 2).

There are many details that still need to be worked out, but the key takeaway messages from the proposed replacement bill are threefold: first, fewer people will have health insurance coverage because the tax credits will be insufficient to induce voluntary purchase, and because states will have less money and be forced to roll back Medicaid coverage. Second, the premiums and cost-sharing contributions of low-income Americans will increase sharply, not only because the plan eliminates cost-sharing subsidies but also because insurers would be allowed to sell catastrophic plans with high cost-sharing requirements. Third, the financing to pay for all expenditures associated with the replacement plan (e.g., the tax credits) will be far more regressive given the repeal of taxation on wealthy Americans. In stark contrast to the ACA, these coverage reforms will move the country toward greater health *inequities* and, as such, will exacerbate existing health disparities.

In addition to the coverage reforms, the bill also would eliminate the Prevention and Public Health Fund. This would mean a reduction of at least $1 billion per year in public health funding (based on the last two years

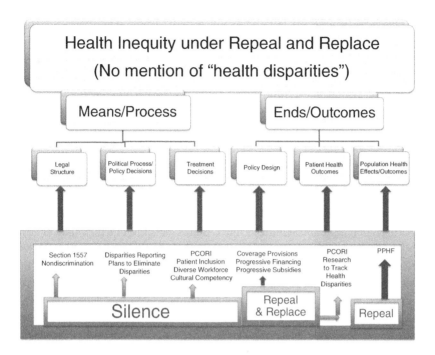

Figure 2 Health Inequity under Repeal and Replace

of appropriations), since the bill specifies no replacement. Local and state health departments would suffer enormously at a time when investment in basic public health infrastructure is arguably already too low, especially in light of ongoing threats of bioterrorism and difficulties in maintaining healthy local environments. Chrissie Juliano, director of the Big Cities Health Coalition (BCHC), a membership organization of twenty-eight urban governmental public health departments, reported: "I cannot underscore the importance of these funds enough . . . . [These funds are] essential to core public health programs that keep Americans healthy and safe every day . . . supporting disease tracking, access to immunizations for those most in need, and preventing and addressing lead poisoning, among other priorities" (Juliano 2017).

The absence of any mention of "health disparities" in the replacement bill is also deafening. While there is no reference to Section 1557 that disallows discrimination, or to any of the provisions calling for reporting on health disparities or creating a plan to eliminate disparities, or to the continued funding for PCORI, most of the changes apply to the coverage provisions—how do we implement better reporting on health disparities when more people are left out of the system? There were new expectations for addressing health disparities, for example, under the Medicaid expansion, but with expansion curtailed, efforts to address health disparities also would go away. While the incentives for delivery model reforms, which also emphasized reducing disparities, will hopefully remain intact, the lack of any mention of a goal to reduce health disparities sets forth a strong signal that the health equity goal that was clearly emphasized in the ACA is no longer valued.

Perhaps of greatest concern is the underlying philosophy of the repeal and replace proposal that so clearly is at odds with moving toward greater health equity. Although the ACA never achieved universal coverage (undocumented immigrants were excluded from the ACA due to another contentious partisan debate), it brought the United States closer to this goal than at any other time in American history, owing to the belief that all Americans deserve access to health care coverage regardless of their circumstances. In striking contrast, the repeal and replace proposal takes us back to beliefs espoused in 1965 when Medicare and Medicaid were enacted—that only certain people are deserving of health care coverage: the elderly under Medicare; the "truly deserving" aged, blind, and disabled under Medicaid; and those who cannot work—under Medicaid. The rest of the population should purchase private health insurance with their earnings. The assumption then was that if one were working, private health insurance would be affordable. That has never been true, and is even less so today. But, for those promoting the replacement bill, it remains their core belief. They want to place the blame for lack of coverage back onto the individual, and remove any sense of public or communal obligation to make sure that everyone has access to health care coverage. If that is truly the belief structure for the new American Health Care Act (if passed by Congress), then we are, sadly and pitifully, moving very far away from achieving health equity.

■ ■ ■

Colleen M. Grogan is a professor at the University of Chicago and academic director of the Graduate Program in Health Administration and Policy (GPHAP). Her research interests include health policy and health politics, the American welfare state, and participatory decision-making processes. She has written several book chapters, articles, and a co-authored book on the history and current politics of the US Medicaid program. She is currently working on a book titled *America's Hidden Health Care State*, which examines the intent behind America's submerged health care state. She is the former editor of the *Journal of Health Politics, Policy and Law*. cgrogan@uchicago.edu

References

APHA (American Public Health Association). 2017. Key ACA Resources. "APHA Fact Sheet: The Prevention and Public Health Fund." www.apha.org/~/media /files/pdf/factsheets/160127_pphf.ashx.

CDC (Centers for Disease Control). Division of Community Health (DCH): Making Healthy Living Easier. "Community Transformation Grants (2011–2014)." www .cdc.gov/nccdphp/dch/programs/communitytransformation/ (accessed on March 7, 2017).

Committee for a Responsible Federal Budget. 2017. "JCT: ACA Repeal Will Cut Taxes by at least $600 Billion." www.crfb.org/blogs/jct-aca-repeal-will-cut-taxes -least-600-billion.

Dorn, Stan, Bowen Garrett, and John Holahan. 2014. "Redistribution under the ACA is Modest in Scope." Urban Institute. www.urban.org/sites/default/files/publication /22271/413023-redistribution-under-the-aca-is-modest-in-scope.pdf.

Fiscella, Kevin. 2011. "Health Care Reform and Equity: Promise, Pitfalls, and Pre-scriptions." *Annals of Family Medicine*, 9: 78–84.

Grogan, Colleen M. 2015. "The Role of the Private Sphere in US Healthcare Enti-tlements: Increased Spending, Weakened Public Mobilization, and Reduced Equity. *Forum* 13, no. 1: 119–42.

"Health Policy Brief: Premium Tax Credits." *Health Affairs*, August 1, 2013.

Juliano, Chrissie. 2017. "ACA Repeal Would Mean Massive Cuts to Public Health, Leaving Cities and States at Risk." *Health Affairs Blog* (March 7). healthaffairs .org/blog/2017/03/07/aca-repeal-would-mean-massive-cuts-to-public-health-leaving -cities-and-states-at-risk/.

Mermin, Gordon B. 2017. "The Big Tax Changes in the House GOP Health Plan." Tax Policy Center: Urban Institute and Brookings Institution. www.taxpolicycenter.org /taxvox/big-tax-changes-house-gop-health-plan.

Park, Edwin, Aviva Aron-Dine, and Matt Broaddus. 2017. "House Republican Health Plan Shifts $370 Billion in Medicaid Costs to States." Center on Budget and Policy Priorities. Website: www.cbpp.org/research/health/house-republican-health-plan -shifts-370-billion-in-medicaid-costs-to-states.

Pollack, Harold. 2011. "Prevention and Public Health." *Journal of Health Politics, Policy and Law* 36, no. 3: 515–20.

Rice, Thomas. 2011. "A Progressive Turn of Events." *Journal of Health Politics, Policy and Law* 36, no. 3: 491–94.

Watson, Sidney D. "Section 1557 of the Affordable Care Act: Civil Rights, Health Reform, Race, and Equity." *Howard Law Journal* 55, no. 3: 855–85.

Commentary

Health Equity in a Trump Administration

Deborah Stone
Brandeis University

Abstract Donald Trump's rhetoric and leadership are destroying the "culture of community" necessary for progress on health equity. His one-line promises to provide "quality health care at a fraction of the cost" smack of neoliberal nostrums that shifted ever more costs onto patients, thereby preventing many people from getting care. The dangers of Trump go far beyond health policy, however; Trump's presidency threatens the political and cultural institutions that make any good policy possible.

Keywords Trump, health equity, health care

The authors of this special issue on health equity wrote their articles at a time when a Trump victory was unthinkable. Although they were able to make some revisions after the election, the editors thought the issue needed at least a short piece written with the knowledge of a Trump administration as a *fait accompli*, and that is the charge they gave me: What might a Trump administration mean for health equity?

I accepted the charge reluctantly, partly because prognostication one month into a cataclysmic political shift is a fool's errand, but mostly because I knew that having to write about this nightmare would force me out of denial and my own self-imposed news ban. When I shared those reasons with Colleen Grogan, the journal's outgoing editor, she said, "I hear you, but I find it helps to write." I don't know whether the pen is mightier than the Tweet or whether reason can triumph over rage, but Colleen reminded me that the antidote to despair is fighting back.

Journal of Health Politics, Policy and Law, Vol. 42, No. 5, October 2017
DOI 10.1215/03616878-3940517   © 2017 by Duke University Press

In that spirit, I will discuss health care in this commentary, because this is a journal about health policy, but I can't emphasize enough that Americans will lose the war for survival as a political community if we allow Trump to pick us off one policy battle at a time—now health care, now education, now work and wages, now climate change, now science, now media. Thus, I try to frame health care in the context of the bigger questions of what we're fighting for and what we're fighting against. We are fighting for equity in health care, yes, but far more urgently for the ideal of equality for all people and for repair of our broken constitutional democracy. We're fighting against a president and a servile Republican Party bent on fomenting hatred and conflict in order to destroy the American social compact and the rule of law. Trump's behavior during the campaign and since his inauguration have violated not only the norms and rules of American politics, but even the pretense of caring about norms and rules. While we all continue to fight for health equity, let's keep foremost in our minds that we're fighting to preserve equality as a political aspiration and rule of law as our way of conducting public life.

Why use the term "health equity" instead of "equality"? We use the term equity to mean, loosely, treating everyone fairly, and, in this loose sense, it differs from how people generally understand equality. Equality denotes sameness. Intuitively, equal opportunity suggests that everyone has exactly the same chance to fulfill their goals. The dilemma of equality is that giving everyone their fair share or an equal crack at personal success often means—and *should* mean—giving people unequal shares or treating them differently on account of differences among them that seem important. Equity, then, denotes a distribution that treats people differently for good reasons, reasons people agree are legitimate. Nowhere is this idea more obvious than in health. Equal access to care or equal medical treatment does not mean "one person, one hip replacement." It means each person should get the medical procedures appropriate, necessary, and effective for his or her illnesses.

Without saying so explicitly, most health policy scholars assume this principle of distribution according to medical need. They assume that no standard other than medical need—not race, gender, age, national origin, sexual orientation, or religion—ought to influence whether people receive medical care or what kinds of care they get. When distribution of medical care seems to be correlated with these nonmedical factors, the apparent deviation from a medical need standard is often taken as evidence of discrimination. The medical need standard also dictates that place of residence should not have a strong influence on whether people receive adequate care. Even though public health and welfare are matters of state responsibility, the medical need standard would seem to be violated when there are large differences in access to care across states or across smaller areas within states. Equity in health also means that in so far as the burdens of illness and disability are preventable or can be lessened through medical care and other human interventions, they should not be correlated with race, gender, age, national origin, sexual orientation, or religion.

Importantly, equity is a political aspiration even more than it is a philosophical or technical standard for evaluating distributive justice. As a political aspiration, equity can be sustained only by a culture of community. Donald Trump threatens equity most gravely not by the specific policies his government will likely enact, but by his vigorous attacks on the culture of community.

What is a culture of community? First, in a culture of community, people are disposed to see the similarities among members of the community more than the differences. Or, put another way, the members believe they share some kind of abiding sameness, a sameness that has overarching importance to how the polity treats its individual members. In the case of health, it goes without saying that there is huge variation in health status and therefore medical need, but the abiding sameness resides in an understanding that we are all biological creatures, vulnerable to disease and disability, and that good health is a prerequisite to every other kind of opportunity and pursuit that people desire.

Second, a culture of community means that people are willing—and actively want—to help other members of their community because they understand that individuals sometimes encounter problems they can't overcome themselves, and they understand the power of collective action and mutual aid. This is the cultural attitude that underlies risk-sharing and insurance.

Third, a culture of community means that people are willing to differentiate among members of the community for all kinds of purposes, yet they have some shared understanding of what they consider legitimate bases and purposes for differentiating. Thus, for example, hiring and promotion decisions, college admissions, and yes, selection for political office, should be based on merit, not on a lottery that gives everyone a strictly equal statistical chance of success. And access to medical care should be based on the need for care, not on ability to pay, and not (as in the Oregon Medicaid program) on a lottery.

Presidents lead with rhetoric as much as they lead with their policy goals. Make no mistake: Donald Trump intends his poisonous rhetoric to change what will be considered the legitimate bases for differentiating among people in public policies. Trump campaigned by strategically cultivating division and resentment. He deliberately nurtured animosity based on race, religion, immigration status, and nationality as a way to gain the political support of groups whose agendas, if not also motives, are to denigrate and suppress women, blacks, Jews, Muslims, immigrants, and LGBT people. As president, he continues to portray the world in terms of "them versus us": immigrants versus natives, terrorists versus Americans, other countries—including our trading partners and NATO allies—versus America, Muslims versus Christians, and his enemies versus him. By accepting the endorsements of White Nationalists and other members and supporters of hate groups, and by appointing high officials who share his hostilities, Trump has all but declared racism, misogyny, homophobia, anti-Semitism, nativism, and xenophobia to be national policy. He has appointed a secretary of education who will do everything in her power to further destroy public schools as vehicles for common socialization and integration. This overall attack on the culture of community will undermine support for universal health insurance, but before I turn to describing how, let me come back to Ground Zero: everyone should be fighting for the larger culture of equity, not merely equity in specific policy areas.

In the United States, the idea of a right to health care never put down enough roots to grow the strong institutions that sustain universal health insurance elsewhere. I've always been mystified why some people think that having government guarantee them access to medical care *diminishes* their personal well-being, while owning a gun increases it. Of course I know the answer, but it's still a mystery. Such people understand all too well that most of what people pay in insurance premiums or taxes goes to pay for people who need medical care more than they do. In other words, when you buy insurance, until you wind up in a hospital you can tell yourself that you're paying for other people. In a culture that nourishes a sense of them versus us and preaches responsibility for oneself, insurance is a hard sell. So is the concept of medical need. "They wouldn't need medical care if they were more responsible and behaved better."

Along comes a president who espouses the self-made man as reality rather than image and believes he is one. A president who can't fathom that everyone gets to where they are thanks to help from family and friends, and from the schools, hospitals, stable banking systems, and legal protections that their society provides for them. A president who gains his political support from people who believe, as one man at a Trump rally said, "The white working class [are] the ones paying for all the others." The man continued, "Finally, we're getting someone who'll do something about it" (quoted in Danner 2016: 8). Trump gives voice to—or rather, shrieks to— the racial, class, nativist, and sexist resentments that make risk-pooling appear wrong and harmful, and that make it morally imperative (so his supporters believe) to dismantle the Affordable Care Act (ACA), Medicare, and Medicaid as much as politically possible.

Arguably, the ACA's most important achievement was to prohibit insurers from denying coverage to people who have "preexisting conditions." In plain English, that clunky phrase means people who are sick or might get sick (woe to them and their families), and thereby cause their insurer to have to pay big medical bills on their behalf (woe to the insurer's profit). Until President Bill Clinton's drive for national health insurance, *preexisting condition* was a piece of technical insurance jargon that commercial insurers used to disguise their core business strategy of refusing to insure sick people (Stone 1993). By now, though, politicians, media, and ordinary people use this once-arcane term as a synonym for sickness or disability. Underneath all the talk of repealing Obamacare, there remains almost universal support for keeping its prohibition on preexisting conditions—by which people don't mean banning sickness itself, but prohibiting insurers from refusing to insure sick people or charging them significantly higher premiums.

This ambiguity of the term *preexisting condition* in popular discourse might actually help the cause of broad risk-pooling. Because *preexisting condition* makes no mention of illness, it takes the focus away from a causal story that holds sick people to blame for their illness, and instead points the finger at insurers who deny sick people coverage. A preexisting condition sounds more like a fact of nature or an act of God than a behavior or character trait for which individuals can be held responsible. The same people who oppose "paying for all the others" want to preserve the ban on preexisting condition denials, yet they don't understand that such a ban promotes precisely the risk-pooling they abhor.

What a delicious irony: a piece of insurance industry jargon meant to disguise discrimination against sick people has become the weapon sick people use to force insurers to do what they're supposed to do—help sick people get medical care. When I told friends I was writing about health care under Trump, a few asked me if I could give them a ray of hope. Well, here's a small one. But it's only small, and it's very fragile. Even if a federal legislative brake on outright coverage denials remains in place, we should scrutinize how insurers continue to squeeze out sick people by manipulating provider networks, benefit packages, and drug formularies, and by strategic marketing.

As I write this commentary, so far Trump's only proposal for health reform smells and tastes like snake oil: "We're going to have great health care at a fraction of the cost, and you watch. It'll happen." That's a line he repeated nearly verbatim at rallies, and again in his speech announcing Tom Price as his choice for secretary of the Department of Health and Human Services (HHS). We can deride his fatuous promises or the gullible people taken in by them, but it's a sobering thought that Trump's oil is only a less refined version of the neoliberal nostrums both parties have peddled for the last forty years.

Consider how Alain Enthoven, the intellectual godfather of managed care, summarized his blueprint for health reform in 1978: "Cutting Cost without Cutting the Quality of Care." That was the title of his "Shattuck Lecture" featured in the prestigious *New England Journal of Medicine* (Enthoven 1978). Enthoven and others elaborated this menu for a free lunch in a series of articles and policy documents, all promising people more freedom to purchase exactly the care they needed and wanted, while in fact reducing their choices and their benefits. To take one example, Medicare Advantage plans indeed reduce up-front premiums compared to traditional Medicare, but people in the Advantage plans pay much higher cost-sharing if they actually use care, and their choice of providers is far more restricted.

Thus, Trump's populist sleight-of-hand is nothing new, but his crass packaging of what has become the essential direction of American health policy does expose the hypocrisy at the center of it all. To the extent that liberals have been acquiescing in this neoliberal fantasy in hopes of achieving some incremental advances in equity, they might have gained a bit of ground here and there, but, on the whole, they bought a pig in a poke. Managed care cuts costs by churning people in and out of plans, disrupting doctor-patient relationships, and forcing people with limited means to choose between medical care and other life necessities. Reductions in government spending indeed reduce the cost of medical care *to govern-ment*, but no matter how you slice it, they also reduce the volume and quality of care for individuals. The one form of spending reduction that might improve quality and equitable distribution would be price controls on drugs and hospitals. That is not on Trump's or Congress's menu.

What about policies that disproportionately harm — and some would say discriminate against — blacks, women, people with disabilities, and people with low incomes? As Mark Hall points out in his article in this issue, most of the major advances against discrimination in health care over the last sixty years have not resulted from court decisions, but rather from regulations issued by administrative agencies and from administrative interpretations of statutes and regulations. In all areas of discrimination law, courts have moved away from the standard of "disparate impact," the potent legal tool developed in the early 1970s to attack actions and policies that might not be explicitly discriminatory—"no blacks, women, etc., allowed"—but that exclude and harm particular categories of people nonetheless. More and more, however, courts require plaintiffs in antidiscrimination cases to prove that a policy maker *intended* to discriminate against them. Here's another ray of hope: normally, proving intentional discrimination is next-to-impossible, but Trump, thanks to his lack of filters, may be making it easier.

The Affordable Care Act includes the strongest antidiscrimination provisions of any health legislation (in Section 1557). Under President Obama's administration, the HHS implementing regulations went a long way toward restoring the disparate impact standard by specifically authorizing private plaintiffs to bring disparate impact claims (see Hall, this issue). Given the Trump administration's intent to dismantle the ACA and all of its regulations, we can expect it to undo much of what progress has been made in restraining the actions of medical providers and insurers that disproportionately harm blacks, women, people with disabilities, and people with low incomes.

There's a lot more to be said about the future of health equity, and think tanks and scholars are already saying it in detailed analyses of Republican proposals, for example, to convert Medicaid to a state block grant program and to replace comprehensive insurance with catastrophic coverage only. Women's advocacy groups such as the Center for Reproductive Rights have carefully calculated what overturning *Roe v. Wade* and defunding Planned Parenthood will mean. The health equity terrain looks mighty rough, but the general political terrain looks even more devastated.

Despite the media's best efforts to portray Trump's inauguration as a "smooth and peaceful transition of power," his administration launched in explosive chaos, with an executive order on immigration that three appellate court judges politely laughed out of court, and with the president seeking to discredit judges who rule against him. It's clear that Trump will continue to use his bully pulpit to undermine the legitimacy of all American political institutions except the presidency he now holds. Trump's targets may include elections, courts, regulatory agencies within the executive branch, and perhaps Congress if, at some point, one or both houses do not buckle to his will. He will continue to undermine the legitimacy of the cultural institutions on which progress and democracy depend—science, news media, and reasoned debate. And he will continue to undermine the rule of law—the one institution that distinguishes the so-called advanced countries from places where violence, coercion, and corruption are the everyday means of conducting collective life.

All of us concerned for the future of American government, prosperity, and well-being, not to mention the well-being of people everywhere in the world and of Planet Earth, had best broaden our concerns for specific policy areas to attend to the survival of US democracy. Yes, we need to put up resistance in every policy corner where Trump and his policies are going to cause havoc and suffering. We need to resist in small places and small ways everywhere. But let's also keep our minds and our energies on the political and cultural institutions that make good policy possible at all.

February 13, 2017

∎ ∎ ∎

Deborah Stone is currently a distinguished visiting professor in the Heller School for Social Policy and Management at Brandeis University. She is the author of four books and numerous articles on health care and social policy.
Stone@brandeis.edu

References

Danner, Mark. 2016. "The Real Trump." Review of *Trump Revealed: An American Journey of Ambition, Ego, Money, and Power*, by Michael Kranish and Marc Fisher. *New York Review of Books* 43, no. 20: 8–14.

Enthoven, Alain C. 1978. "Shattuck Lecture: Cutting Cost without Cutting the Quality of Care." *New England Journal of Medicine* 298: 1229–38.

Stone, Deborah. 1993. "The Struggle for the Soul of Health Insurance." *Journal of Health Politics, Policy and Law* 18, no. 2: 287–317.

Printed and bound by CPI Group (UK) Ltd, Croydon, CR0 4YY

09/06/2025

14685756-0001